A Diagnosis for Our Times

SUNY series in the Sociology of Culture
Charles R. Simpson, editor

A Diagnosis for Our Times

Alternative Health, from Lifeworld to Politics

Matthew Schneirov
Jonathan David Geczik

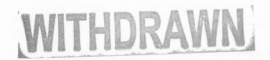

State University Press of New York

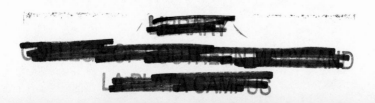

Published by
State University of New York Press, Albany

For information, address State University of New York Press,
90 State Street, Suite 700, Albany, NY 12207

Production by Kelli Williams
Marketing by Jennifer Giovani

Library of Congress Cataloging-in-Publication-Data

Schneirov, Matthew.
  A diagnosis for our times: alternative health, from lifeworld to politics / Matthew
Schneirov, Jonathan David Geczik.
    p. cm.—(SUNY series in sociology of culture)
  Includes bibliographical and references and index.
  ISBN 0-7914-5731-1 (hbk.: alk. paper)—ISBN 0-7914-5732-X (pbk.: alk. paper)
  1. Alternative medicine 2. Social medicine. I. Geczik, Jonathan David II. Title. III.
Series.

R733 .S366 2003
615.5—dc21
                                                                    2002042635

10 9 8 7 6 5 4 3 2 1

To Jon whose passion for life and learning made this all possible and to Rebecca, who loves books.

Contents

Acknowledgments

This book was truly a product of a joint effort of my colleague and friend, Jonathan David Geczik and myself. We began with the same curiosity and excitement about our research but with somewhat different assessments of where it would lead. We often argued, with varying degrees of intensity, over how to assess and interpret our data. Years later, after traveling throughout the Western Pennsylvania area doing interviews, going to meetings, attending lectures and the like and then discussing what we saw and heard, we developed an almost identical orientation toward our subject. In fact, by the last few chapters, we would compose together, and finish one another's sentences. Jon's keen intellect, passion for life and learning, as well as his immersion in the alternative health community really made this whole project possible from the beginning. His untimely death, the same day the SUNY editorial board voted to publish our manuscript, left me and his many other friends in a state of shock, which still continues. This book is part of the legacy Jon leaves to loved ones, friends, and I hope to many others.

I would also like to thank the many colleagues at Duquesne University who offered advice and support. Doug Harper, Richard Colignon, Charles Hanna, and Fred Evans provided useful criticisms and suggestions. The Social and Public Policy Center and its director Mike Irwin provided graduate research assistants, help with transcriptions and useful technical assistance while Duquesne University's internal grants allowed me to spend summers doing research. Many colleagues commented on early drafts of various chapters at regional and national sociology conferences, and we incorporated many of these comments and criticisms into the final draft. Thanks to John Markoff, Sidney Tarrow, and David Eisenberg for their encouragement and special thanks to Norm Denzin and Joseph Kotarba who read various sections of this manuscript in an early form and helped to shape the final product. Greg Field and Robert Johnston, two historians interested in alternative health, provided encouragement and helpful comments. Editors and reviewers at SUNY press saw the potential in this work and helped us to correct some of its limitations.

One of the pleasures of doing fieldwork is the opportunity it presents to meet people who can change your life for the better. Many of these people we refer to in the text, the founder and leader of Holistic Living Quest, the chair of the Committee for Freedom of Choice in Cancer Therapy, the director of Whole Health Resources, a prominent holistic physician, managers of a health store, an impressive young woman struggling with Hepatitis C, and many others, too numerous to mention. So many times in doing interviews we were so stimulated and fascinated by these conversations, that and John and I would spend hours afterward talking about what we had learned. By and large the alternative health community welcomed us and invited us to participate in virtually all their activities. To all our friends in this community, we offer our thanks. Special thanks to the leadership of the UPMC Complementary Medicine Clinic for providing us with so much information and for opening the clinic and its staff to us. Of course, we offer special thanks to the folks who graciously agreed to be interviewed.

The author and publisher are grateful to the following for permission to use previously published material in this book:

Matthew Schneirov and Jonathan David Grecik, "A Diagnosis for Our Times: Alternative Health's Submerged Networks and the Transformation of Identities."
Copyright 1996 by the Midwest Sociological Society
Reprinted from *The Sociological Quarterly*
Vol. 37. No. 4. by permission of the University of California Press

Matthew Schneirov and Jonathan David Grecik, "Technologies of the Self and the Aesthetic Project of Alternative Health."
Copyright 1998 by the Midwest Sociological Society
Reprinted from *The Sociological Quarterly*
Vol. 39. No. 3. by permission of the University of California Press

Matthew Schneirov and Jonathan David Grecik, "Alternative Health and the Challenges of Institutionalization."
Health: An Interdisciplinary Journal of the Social Study of Health, Illness, and Medicine.
Vol. 6. No. 2., pp. 201–220. Reprinted by permission of Sage Publications Ltd. © Sage Publications Ltd., 2002.

Finally, family and friends were a constant source of encouragement. My cousin, Mark Wolynn, now a prominent alternative health practitioner, began his career when this research was first beginning. The hours of discussions, access to information about some of his patients, and free sessions helped me to clarify many ideas and feel better! Mary Beth Belsito, a good friend, was enthusiastic about the project and provided many insights. Dena Vrabel, a massage therapist and friend, first introduced me to a physician in the Complementary Medicine Clinic and helped to get this phase of the research going. Dr. Vered Lewy, my wife's cousin, commented on portions of the manuscript and provided some technical assistance on medical issues. My wife Shari, who taught me much about herbal tea and the pleasures of eating organic greens, is the source of what is most healthy about my life.

Introduction

Two Vignettes

Arthur Sutton is a part-time accountant who is also the founder of an organization called Holistic Living Quest (HLQ), a loosely organized collective that disseminates information on alternative health, grassroots social activism, and various Eastern and New Age forms of spirituality. Monthly mailings are sent to a list of people and the group also sponsors events such as a yearly awards banquet for people who had distinguished themselves in these efforts. HLQ also sponsors a range of activities called Wellness 2000, an effort to link alternative health with other social movements not ordinarily associated with alternative health—the labor movement, religious progressives, and the ecology movement, for example. In addition, Wellness 2000 is engaged in efforts to enhance the legitimacy of alternative health through establishing an HMO and by seeking health insurance coverage.

How does an accountant become a full-time alternative health activist and a founder of an organization that coordinates alternative health activities? Art began his journey in the 1970s after his divorce to his first and only wife, Chris. Around this time Art began to explore his own attitudes toward women, his spirituality, and self-help groups that focused on personal growth and self-examination. He decided to leave Pittsburgh and traveled through Europe and the Middle East in a spiritual quest to redefine his life and seek an ultimate purpose. He traveled

1

to India, Israel, Greece, and Scotland where he met a variety of mentors who enlightened him about a number of religious and spiritual traditions. When Art returned to the United States he enrolled in a New Thought theology school in California and lived communally for thirteen months. During this time Art had a mystical experience during a Gestalt workshop where "the gates opened up to a higher reality."

While becoming interested in telepathy, precognition, and Eastern spiritual practices, Art solidified his belief that "disease is an expression of a fixation in certain behavior patterns." In other words, for Art, when people become frozen in repetitive habits that assert a monopoly over their lives, disease manifests itself. Critical in this respect is money for, as Art is fond of saying, "money is the most habitual habit we're stuck on." As a result Art is able to link his training in accounting with his interest in health and spirituality for "money is the most emotional thing there is" and because of that the most dangerous to health. Approaching an almost postmodern sensibility, Art advocates a fluid, open stance toward experience where emotions and beliefs are never allowed to become closed boundaries capturing the person within them. HLQ can be conceived of as an organizational arena that attempts to break through narrow boundaries of thought and emotion.

Eventually Art decided to move back to Pittsburgh because "he knew he had to return" to bring these insights to the public life of Pittsburgh. He became convinced that "New Age" people with their solipsistic preoccupation with the self could never be a sufficient means to change the world. The view that "I just need to work on myself and the world will change around me" he calls the "New Age cop out." Nevertheless, Art is sympathetic with New Age spirituality and its commitment to self-transformation. Art has strong commitments to the intentional community movement, the men's movement, feminism, ecology, progressive religious groups and more broadly grassroots activism. Art no longer believes in conventional monogamous marriage, would like to have several wives, believes in communal living arrangements, and in living simply with less money. Much of this he has been able to put into practice. He works part time and earns only enough to maintain a relatively simple lifestyle, despite being in a profession that if pursued full time would allow him to live much more comfortably.

Ed Watkowsky is also an alternative health activist but couldn't be more different from Art. Ed, a regular at his local Methodist Church, is one of the organizers of the Committee for Freedom of Choice in

Cancer Therapy (CFC). The CFC, which recently held its twenty-year anniversary, holds monthly meetings that introduce to an audience of middle-aged and elderly people a range of alternative treatments for cancer and other diseases. Literature is displayed, videos are shown, organic food is sold, and guest speakers representing a wide range of alternative health care modalities are brought in to speak each month. Ed has lived in a small town bordering Pittsburgh all his life, where he was a steelworker and member of the USW. He has since retired and now spends most of his time advocating the cause of alternative health, and inventing and promoting his own water purification system.

Ed has been married most of his life to the same woman, Sandra. He says he married Sandra because he "got her pregnant" and it was the right thing to do. Unlike couples who "fall in love" and then "ten weeks later they're trying to make out with someone else," Ed has grown closer to Sandra over the years and they work together (she works in a health food store) and share the same religious values and commitment to alternative health. Ed's daughter is estranged from him because she had a child out of wedlock. Despite the urging of his friends to reconcile with her, Ed cannot because he believes that his daughter needs to acknowledge her sin before he can forgive her.

Many years ago Ed was introduced to alternative medicine through his good friends Tom and Ellen. Ellen had been diagnosed with breast cancer and her health was rapidly deteriorating. As devout Christians both couples believed in the power of prayer. As Ed put it, "We were praying. Lord your will be done." Ed thought that only prayer could heal Ellen after she had tried chemotherapy, radiation, and a number of operations without success. If she did not recover, it "was God's will." But one day Ed and Sandra bumped into Tom and Ellen at the local Eat and Park restaurant and discovered that Tom had become an advocate of alternative cancer treatments and had convinced Ellen to try these unconventional treatments. It was Ed's friend Tom who envisioned a new organization that would provide support for cancer patients seeking alternatives to conventional treatments for cancer.

Shortly after, Ed became instrumental in the formation of the CFC and, as he put it, "the word spread through a local radio interview and through word of mouth." Originally the group was loosely affiliated with support groups for a California doctor who was in danger of losing his license for using unauthorized and "dangerous" alternative treatments for cancer (laetrile). While this case has long been resolved, the CFC remains in existence and now focuses on its original mission of supplying information, networking, and support for people seeking alternative treatments for cancer and other chronic diseases.

For Ed alternative health is no peripheral matter. It is his life's work, so much so that he was regarded as a pariah in his church and this causes him anguish and grief. Alternative health, as Ed puts it, is still associated with dark and satanic forces by some members of his own church, despite its roots in many evangelical congregations. Ed believes strongly in voluntarism and self-help, departing from the welfare state liberalism that was part of his working-class roots. Many of his positions on social and cultural issues are conservative with a dollop of libertarianism. For example, he personally opposes abortion but is also against the state prohibiting it. Instead, he believes that a woman who receives an abortion should be "shunned" by the community.

How did Art and Ed, coming from such disparate social backgrounds with distinct biographies and world views, come to forge a common commitment to alternative health? This is a complex issue that will be explored throughout the book but for now we can see that it points to the fact that alternative health slices through traditional boundaries between the political Right and Left, conservatism and liberalism. These two people also illustrate an unexpected convergence at another level—the body that provides a source for new orientations and sensibilities that are still in the process of crystallization.

The Study of Two Health Networks

Art and Ed are activists in two distinct alternative health networks. While both pursue their health commitments in geographical proximity to one another, they inhabit distinctly different worlds. Art is likely to converse with astrologers, goddess worshipers, mystics and channelers, participants in various men's movements, ecology activists, and local radicals engaged in community organizing. Art floats back and forth comfortably among all of these groups—both cultural experimenters, political radicals, and the strange and eccentric. His home is a communal gathering point for all these groups. This is not a temporary episode but the core commitment and identity in Art's life.

Ed would not be comfortable in these circles. From the point of view of an observer, his life would be conventional for a working-class man in a small town. When we talked to Ed at his home, his wife Sandra was present but said little except to affirm her husband's many opinions and observations. Ed told us about his life as a steelworker, his traditional views about family, sexuality, religion, and politics. Yet when the discussion shifted to health Ed sounded a lot like Art. Both believe that the individual is responsible for his or her health and should be free to explore modalities, including experimental approaches, independent of government regulation. Both criticized the medical establishment for enforcing a regimen that had limited effectiveness against a range of chronic illnesses and that ignored the spiritual dimension of health and illness. Both also expressed a commitment to voluntarism and community rather than government regulation and bureaucratically administered care. Because of his commitment to alternative health his minister and fellow parishioners ostracized him and criticized his commitments.

It was easy to find out about Art and his HLQ activities for they published an alternative health directory sold at the local food co-op. We contacted as many of the practitioners who advertised in this directory as we could, trying to interview representatives of a range of alternative health modalities. In many cases were able to interview some of the clients or "patients" of these practitioners who told us about the way they cope with illness and their experiences with conventional doctors and in alternative health. Eventually we were invited to attend meetings of Wellness 2000, and special events sponsored by HLQ. Our contacts with many in this community provided us with the opportunity to invite some of them to a number of focus groups where we discussed a range of issues.

At the same time, we heard through word of mouth about a group concerned with alternative cancer treatments that met in a town north of Pittsburgh. We started to attend their monthly meetings and through this we introduced ourselves to Ed and other regular participants. Through these contacts we learned about a closely related group, the Natural Living Group (NLG). This group sponsors lectures, which emphasize nutrition and sustainable agriculture as well as alternative medicine, and has been meeting regularly since 1958. The NLG originally functioned as an organic food cooperative providing members with fresh organic fruits and vegetables. It no longer operates as a food co-op and instead sponsors weekly lectures on alternative nutrition and health care and sponsors a yearly food festival. Today meetings consist of between eighty and one hundred people, most of them elderly (in contrast to meetings in the 1960s and 1970s that attracted a range of ages). Speakers at the monthly meetings give talks about "The Fats in Our Lives: Then and Now," "Hypoglycemia, Diabetes and Emotional

Disorders," "Pollution Most Likely Culprit for Latest List of Ills," "Dealing With Candidiasis and Allergies," among many other topics. The speakers are typically advocates of nutritional approaches for maintaining health or for addressing particular health problems. The NLG was part of the Health Foods Movement, which emerged in the 1930s as an alternative approach to the discoveries of nutritional science. In the view of the NLG, food has been "devitalized" or depleted of its minerals and essential nutrients by modern agricultural planting practices and by the application of chemicals—fertilizers, pesticides, and preservatives. The leaders of both the CFC and NLG know one another well and go to each other's meetings but are far less likely to shop at the Pittsburgh co-op or interact with HLQ members. It was more difficult for us to get to know members of these groups, but we did attend the monthly meetings, interview the leadership of both the CFC and NLG and administer a survey at one well-attended CFC meeting.

From our contacts with both groups we learned about a national organization, the National Health Federation (NHF), that functions both as an interest group, a source for information and health referrals, and a sponsor of conferences and health fairs that provide a forum for practitioners, patients, and activists. We attended a number of regional health fairs, conventions, and meetings sponsored by the NHF and talked to the president of the local chapter. At the first conference we attended, there was much discussion about the head of the federation, Dr. Jonathan Wright, and his harassment by the Federal Food and Drug Administration (FDA). His clinic was raided, files were taken, and his practice was closed down for several months. Discussions around this incident led to the venting of considerable anger at the government and fear about the future of alternative health. Concerns were also expressed about government attempts to regulate vitamins in a fashion analogous to the way prescription drugs are regulated.

A local television station features guests from the Christian alternative health community and emphasizes the compatibility of Christianity and alternative health. Maureen Solomon is a popular and frequent guest who also has a regular show where she offers health advice and interviews alternative health practitioners. Solomon is a nationally known figure whose books are widely distributed in health food stores along with her health products. A chiropractor, Martin Gallagher, along with his wife, also has a show, which parallels the form and content of Solomon's show. There is also a radio station that regularly broadcasts a number of programs on alternative health and is loosely associated with some of the founders of the CFC.

We supplemented approximately sixty semi-structured, intensive interviews (between one and four hours each) with ethnographic research in a variety of alternative health settings. The ages of those we interviewed ranged from twenty-two (a college student) to seventy-eight (the founder of the NLG). All but five had attended college and forty-six of the sixty were women.[1] The sample includes practitioners, patients, and activists. The practitioners we interviewed represent a wide range of alternative therapies: naturopathy, Ayurvedic medicine, astrology, homeopathy, traditional acupuncture, gestalt therapy, chiropractic, reiki, therapeutic touch, massage therapy and Shiatsu, biofeedback, energy medicine, past life regression, attitudinal healing, New Thought theology, macrobiotics, bach flower remedies, herbal medicine, among others. We attended meetings, study groups, health fairs and expos, workshops, cooking classes, patient testimonials, and lectures. We also attended on a regular basis meetings of Wellness 2000, the CFC, a macrobiotic study group, and a lecture series at the local food co-op. We held, or participated in, a series of small meetings with between ten and twelve alternative health practitioners and other activists, in which we discussed a series of issues; how participants defined "holistic"; how they became involved in alternative health; their vision of the future; their perception of the relationship between personal transformation and larger social and political change. Overall, fifty-three activists attended, providing an even larger sample of the alternative health community than provided by our interviews. A more detailed account of these groups will be provided in chapter 5 where we discuss alternative health as a social movement. Throughout the early chapters we provide short case studies from a range of sites in both networks and highlight the comparison between the Christian network (the CFC and NLG) and what we call "the holistic health network" (HLQ, the local food co-op, and a number of other New Age–oriented groups).

Over the past year we interviewed staff members and a number of patients at a "complementary medicine" clinic in a major Pittsburgh hospital as well as observing some of the interaction between patients and practitioners. The view from here, where alternative health physicians and practitioners meet regularly with hospital administrators, write grants, and evaluate their protocols is decidedly different from the point of view of activists in the CFC or the NHF. Included in the sample is a holistic M.D. who practices in one of the major Pittsburgh hospitals as well as a holistic M.D. with his own practice, widely recognized as providing an alternative to biomedicine. We also interviewed a nurse who practices therapeutic touch in a hospital setting where she works with a group of specialists as well a wide range of practitioners who have their own practices or who work cooperatively with other alternative practitioners. In addition, we informally consulted with a number of physicians, both specialists and general practitioners, to assess their use of and response to alternative medicine. In this way we tried to capture what it means be an alternative health practitioner, activist, and patient in a variety of institutional settings and from a variety of points of view, from the casual shopper at the local food co-op to a devotee of macrobiotics attending a study group, from an activist working to establish links with other progressive communities to a patient of a holistic physician at a medicine clinic.

It is commonplace now to observe that ethnographic "data" and writing is in part a construction of the ethnographer's vantage point, methodology, and interpretative framework. What kinds of questions are asked or not asked, the settings within which interviews take place, the very impact of the ethnographers' presence (as well as their class, gender, and racial background), all shape the responses that are received and the development of an ethnographic analysis and narrative. We know that alternative health practitioners will say some things to their colleagues that they would not say to us, or that certain kinds of experiences are difficult for people to put into words, especially in front of strangers. An account of the route into alternative health by an activist will more likely than not be filtered through a kind of "party line" narrative that will make one account sound quite similar to another, making it difficult to reconstruct the experiences or the thought processes of people in real time. When people choose certain words, and draw upon certain discourses and narrative forms to express their experiences, they are already interpreting their experiences just as we interpret what they tell us in light of our own research questions, and analytical frameworks. In this light, how can we arrive at some understanding of alternative health that is scientific and rigorous?

We respond to these issues in the following ways. First, we have used as many approaches to gathering information as possible, from interviews in a variety of settings, to participant observation, focus groups, and extensive reading of alternative health literature. This approach, "triangulation," uses one methodology to make up for the weaknesses of another.[2] For example, the artificiality of the interview setting can be balanced with observations of conversations at meetings and interactions at health fairs. What a manager at the co-op says about her customers and the way the store operates can be checked against other accounts as well as our observations of the interactions in the store. Second, our own experiences with various alternative health modalities and regimes helped us to ask people what we hope are the right questions, and to delve more deeply when there seemed to be a gap in their accounts. In experiencing at least part of the process of becoming involved in alternative health we can become sensitive to what is overlooked in the narratives of seasoned activists. Also, many of the people we interviewed we have come to know over a seven-year period in a variety of settings; bumping into them at the food co-op, interviewing them at their offices, hearing them talk to patients, observing them at meetings. We can, as a result, place their responses to interview questions in this larger context. Finally, we shared with most of our subjects various versions of our work. We received useful feedback from some people, correcting some factual inaccuracies and raising other valuable questions. In addition, we summarized our work in various group settings at HLQ meetings and with leaders of the CFC and NLG. The continuous feedback we received gave us some confidence that our own accounts and interpretations bore a close resemblance to those of our subjects or at least were recognizable to our subjects. The picture that emerges is, we believe, a rounded one.

There are also clear limitations to our research. While we immersed ourselves in one corner of the alternative health world, there are others we did not explore, from gay and lesbian networks who are sharing new experimental approaches to treating AIDS, to various forms of folk medicine, to elements of the feminist health movement. While we paid some attention to the casual user of alternative health products, this was not our primary emphasis. Instead, we focused on the activists, both patients and practitioners within the holistic and Christian networks. We are interested in alternative health as a social movement, its connection to other movements, and its impact on participants. As a result, we do not focus on processes of professionalization within various alternative therapies. While we can say little about these issues, or how patients combine alternative and conventional treatments, we have opened up an area for study that has been overlooked thus far in the literature; the politics of alternative health, from everyday life where alternative health often functions as a "cultural laboratory" to institutional recognition and contestation.

It was our good fortune to have engaged in this study during an important period in the re-emergence of alternative health in America. During the decade of the nineties alternative health in Pittsburgh was a beleaguered fringe, existing primarily among activists embedded in subcultures and only beginning to attract widespread interest. By the end of the decade alternative health had achieved considerable institutional recognition. When we started our research, in 1993, alternative health activists in Pittsburgh complained to us of constant harassment by FDA agents, and a general atmosphere of repression on the national level even while anticipating opportunities for growth. But years later, with the opening of new complementary medicine clinics at two major hospitals, favorable publicity, and a host of new alternative health practices, the climate was noticeably more receptive. The local food co-op has doubled its size and a new organic food store is soon to open in the city. There is also much more racial and age diversity among shoppers at health stores and the food co-op. A number of alternative health cooperative practices have opened in the city as well as new and expanded stores that sell health products. These successes have caused some to seek greater professional and institutional recognition while others are still skeptical that the natural remedies and emphasis on self-care in alternative health will ever be entirely compatible with biomedicine.

The possibility of a new form of "medical pluralism" is suggested by the successes achieved by alternative medicine, so much so that many now refer to their approach as "complementary" or "complementary and alternative medicine."[3] We explore the implications of this development through a study of a complementary medicine clinic and through our study of Wellness 2000, an effort on the part of some alternative health activists to forge ongoing connections within this quite diverse and often fragmented community as well as to develop links to other progressive movements. Regular meetings were held in order to develop a common statement of principles and vision for the future. The leader of this effort, Art Sutton, also had the goal of developing contacts with the political Left in the Pittsburgh area, specifically elements of the labor movement, the Thomas Merton Center (Catholic religious Left), and elements of the ecology movement. We were invited to meetings where cultural radicals and political leftists sat uneasily together, generating some fascinating discussions but little basis for an ongoing coalition. This goal, to forge links within the alternative health community and between it and other progressive communities amounts to an effort to reorient alternative health toward social rather than only personal change. The extent to which this effort achieved any success may tell us something about the possibilities and limits of alternative health as a movement.

Illness is not some exotic feature of someone else's culture. It takes on different forms and meanings depending on the larger social and historical context, but illness itself is a human experience. Both of us have had and continue to cope with chronic illnesses, asthma and high blood pressure for one of us and an intestinal disorder for the other. We've both seen conventional M.D.s and one of us was well acquainted with the world of alternative medicine in Pittsburgh prior to engaging in this research project. Indeed, it would have been difficult, if not impossible to obtain many of our interviews and to be invited to attend many of the meetings and study groups without the trust that some degree of sympathy engenders. Moreover, our personal experiences with alternative health regimes, New Age spirituality, the illnesses of friends and family members (one of our mutual friends went to an alternative cancer clinic in Mexico to be treated for colon cancer), sensitized us to the language and experiences of the patients, activists, and practitioners we encountered.

In the end we were changed by the people we met, the meetings we attended, the regimes we tried, the therapies we explored, much like many of the people we write about. For both of us, our experiences in following alternative health regimes have remained an ongoing part of the texture of our lives. In addition, we both look to our respective pasts for sources of meaning, even if this does not provide an all-encompassing world view. For one of us this means an appropriation of Jewish traditions in the spirit of "Jewish renewal" and for the other this involves an effort to keep alive elements of the music and culture of an ethnic working-class neighborhood.

While we partially identify with the goals of alternative health and have remained in contact with both of the networks we studied, we have also come to understand the limitations of alternative health as a new health paradigm or a social movement with transformative potential. In a sense, alternative health does not fully make the journey from lifeworld to politics and we suggest reasons why this is the case. These limitations are explored in subsequent chapters but for now we want to emphasize that this finding was one we experienced as we observed efforts to broaden alternative health's goals and integrate it into the larger health care system.

Thick and Thin Description

There are two dangers that can undermine adequate social science inquiry. On the one hand, analysis can stay close to the self-descriptions of actors, what Geertz called "experience near" concepts (or "thick descriptions").[4] On the other hand, analysis can range beyond local interpretive contexts and link multiple sectors of society in the form of vast and complex theoretical exercises, that is, experience distant or thin descriptions. A social science that is adequate to its object must consistently show linkages between these two levels of conceptualization—experience near and experience distant concepts.[5] Remaining on the level of thick description does not allow actors to understand the range of factors shaping their lives that are not immediately available to their local understanding. Staying on the level of abstract theory or "thin descriptions" presents the danger of social science not being translatable back to the lifeworld of actors and therefore irrelevant for enlightenment and social transformation.

Throughout the text we have employed critical theories that are clearly "experience distant." But, in order to move beyond description, a task done quite well by many others, and in order to advance our goal of exploring alternative health's transformative potential, we utilize the critical theories of Jürgen Habermas, Michel Foucault, Walter Benjamin, and others. In doing so, we realize that we run the risk of producing a narrative that is often interrupted with an analysis rather distant from the local knowledge of participants. But, theory is an indispensable tool in making connections between phenomena allowing the subject matter to become defamilarized in fruitful ways. At the same time, our use of these theories grew out of particular problems and issues that arose from our data. How can we conceptualize the kind of orientation many patients take toward their bodies when engaged in an alternative health regime? Does alternative health contribute to or resist the "medicalization of society"? What is the relationship between alternative health's critique of bureaucratization and commodification and those of other movements? How does the desire to revive elements of the past relate to similar efforts in other movements and throughout society? Making these connections requires a movement to thin description.

We begin with the local context of alternative health groups in the Pittsburgh area and their interpretations of their own practices and activities. At this level of thick description we describe the daily health routines of patients, networks of association, meetings and lectures, and the words and images that health activists mention in their conversations. For example a key word in the lexicon of alternative health is "nature." Natural foods and remedies are recommended. The goal of alternative health regimes is to stimulate the body's natural rhythms and healing capacity. Traditional societies and healing systems are thought to be less manufactured and closer to nature. We also provide accounts of the way participants understand the process of self-care, their paths into alternative health and criticisms of biomedicine and the larger society. In doing so we remain close to the descriptions of actors.

But we also examine the more anonymous contexts that shape the practices of alternative health—from the nature of the medical industrial complex, various levels of institutionalization of alternative medicine, larger social processes such as commodification, and the corporate bureaucratization of health care and more general changes in modern capitalist societies. We explore the connection between alternative health and other social movements, examine alternative health's relationship to the past in the context of broader issues of the relationship between tradition and the modern world, and evaluate efforts to link alternative health with the dominant health care system. Finally, we ask whether alternative health may contribute to a new health care paradigm whose contours are only beginning to become apparent. These processes and connections are "experience distant," not immediately accessible to actors. It is the obligation of social science research to pay attention to these connections, to the relationship between illness and the total social process.

Lifeworld to Politics

The subtitle "from Lifeworld to Politics" is a restatement of this movement from thick to thin descriptions and their linkage to one another. Complementary to this strategy of employing thick and thin descriptions is the tracing of the movement from lifeworld to politics— from the meanings embedded in everyday life to struggles over resources and power. Art's involvement in HLQ and Ed's involvement in CFC were sparked by personal crises, in the one case divorce and in the other the terminal illness of a close friend. They drew upon different frameworks of meaning to make sense of these personal tragedies and to reorganize their lives in the process. Personal change sowed the seeds for new connections with other people from which emerged more formal networks and associations that they took the lead in forming and sustaining. Today CFC informs its members about legislation that has a direct bearing upon the alternative health community and in some cases recommends direct action to alter or transform the political climate. HLQ is forming alliances with environmental and labor groups around issues of ecology and social justice and is organizing an alternative health HMO and lobbying for insurance coverage.

Another example of personal change sowing the seeds for new associations is one young woman whom we interviewed. Ellen found out that Hepatitis C caused her constant fatigue and susceptibility to a variety of illnesses. Since that diagnosis, she received a regimen of interferon which was partially successful but which also resulted in her inability to continue with work and some serious side effects. She began to see a macrobiotic counselor looking for a better solution. Ellen described for us how her life changed as a result of her immersion in the world of alternative health. The demanding practice of her dietary regime combined with regular attendance at a macro-biotic study group as well as the many new friends she made, caused her to reevaluate her life. Her newfound assertiveness with respect to medical authority led to a reexamination of her stance toward authority in general. She began to read popular feminist literature, including Clarrisa Pinkola Estes's *Women Who Run with the Wolves* and Susan Faludi's *Backlash*. She partially distanced herself from her Catholic upbringing, finding a church that was more reflective of her emerging spirituality. She "worked out" and dieted less, realizing that this had become an obsession and diverted her from more important pursuits. She told us that she valued the slower pace of life, her ability to appreciate her daughter, and little things like walks in the park.

A few years after these experiences, Ellen is no longer committed to the rigors of the macrobiotic diet. Her disease fluctuates between periods of remission, when she can lead a normal life, and periods when her liver disease makes life difficult. She still sees her doctor who is treating her with interferon but has retained her commitment to alternative health. The alternative health network she participated in when her disease was first diagnosed is still a resource for her as she struggles to cope with her illness and give it meaning. Her commitment to feminism, sparked by her illness and involvement in alternative health, remains an ongoing part of her life.

Ed's, Art's, and Ellen's experiences are reflective of the growing political potential of existential issues related to illness and health. On the one hand, there is growing disenchantment with conventional medicine and its lack of efficacy in treating a range of chronic health problems. There is also disillusionment with the way the health care system reduces individual responsibility. Finally, the financial burden of conventional medicine and its unsustainable increase in the cost of its treatments stimulates a search for alternatives. On the other hand, the biomedical model is unable to make the transition between its practices and wider horizons of meaning. Illness, especially if it's terminal, becomes senseless when the body is viewed as a machine that is detached from the person's life and relationships. Alternative health, we argue, is a response to the institutional crisis of the health care system and the separation of health care from larger contexts of meaning.

We begin by placing our own work in the larger social context of the rise of chronic disease, and the cultural changes that made the reemergence of alternative health possible. We also provide an overview of other research on alternative health and how our own breaks new ground in examining alternative health as a social movement. Chapter 2 discusses the impact of biomedical hegemony on the problem of meaning in modern societies. When subjected to medical intervention, major life course transitions and crises are no longer encoded in larger cultural horizons. Is this disenchantment of the body the price we pay for the scientific advances of modern medicine? Alternative health, we argue, is an effort to reintegrate effectiveness and enchantment with respect to health and illness. We pay special attention to the problems of biomedicine in mediating its language with the language and practices of patients. Also in this chapter we explore alternative health as an expert system but with a close proximity to the lifeworld. These opening chapters are intended to provide an introduction to chapters 3 through 6 which are based on our research.

In chapter 3 we examine the everyday lives of patients and their encounters with health traditions through their use of alternative health products and their adoption of alternative health protocols. Here patients and activists contextualize their lives in larger horizons of meaning which we comprehend through the concept of reenchantment and Walter Benjamin's conception of the aura. Alternative health patients and activists experience through their practices and use of health products flashes of reconciliation with the past and the natural world. These experiences provide the energy for many to reevaluate their lives and transform their identities.

In chapter 4 we explore the alternative health regime or what we call, following Michel Foucault, "technologies of the self." We argue that patients who participate in this process of self-care are engaging in an aesthetic practice that aims at transforming their lives. We call this the classical aesthetic project, an effort to transform the body and the self so that the person is in a state of harmony with the natural world.

We demonstrate that through these aesthetic practices, patients are step by step made available for political action.

Chapter 5 explores alternative health as a social movement utilizing the new social movement theories of Jürgen Habermas and Alberto Melucci. Here we move from the realm of meaning in the lifeworld to the realm of politics and social action. Alternative health, we argue, constitutes a submerged social movement network and shares with other new social movements a resistance to bureaucratization and partial resistance to commodification. This resistance to bureaucratization and commodification cuts across the commonly understood divide between the political Left and Right. At the level of everyday life we see alternative health as contributing to a value shift, toward what some have called "postmaterial values" and a critique of progress. At the level of discourse and organization, the implications of this value shift are more complex.

Next we examine the fruits of efforts to integrate biomedicine and alternative health through a case study of a complementary medicine clinic at a major hospital. We explore the link between two levels of power in the alternative health movement, the institutional level and alternative health's subculture or what we call "submerged networks." Through interviews and observations with the clinic's staff and patients we ask whether alternative health's growing success in achieving institutional recognition is coming at the price of its submerged networks and core identity.

Finally, we engage in a more global discussion of how alternative health is bound to more general aspects of the total social process, how it is an essential ingredient in the potential emergence of a radically transformed understanding of health and illness, and crucial for the formation of a new politics of health.

The Study of Alternative Health

In a study in the *New England Journal of Medicine,* researchers discovered that Americans spent nearly $11.7 billion on alternative health treatments in 1990, much of which was out of pocket. These treatments included chiropractic, massage therapy, homeopathy, lifestyle diets, among other approaches. Most patients used unconventional approaches along with more conventional allopathic treatments but rarely told their doctors that they were seeing an alternative practitioner. Overall, one in three Americans in 1990 reported using at least one unconventional therapy in the past year and one-third of these saw providers for unconventional therapy. Use of unconventional treatments was more prevalent among those with some college education, contesting any simple equation between alternative health practices and lack of sophistication about the modern world. In a follow-up study, seven years later, researchers found even greater interest in alternative health. In 1997, 42 percent reported using an alternative therapy and over the seven-year period from the first study there was a 47.3 percent growth in the number of visits made to alternative practitioners.[1]

A Bill Moyers PBS series (and best-selling book) explored sympathetically a variety of unconventional treatments for chronic diseases,[2] and this series has spawned a number of CNN and other special documentaries on alternative medicine. At the same time, books presenting holistic and alternative approaches to health from Dean Ornish[3] and Andrew Weil[4] to Depak Chopra[5] have made the *New York*

Times best-sellers list. On the legislative front an effort by the Federal Food and Drug Administration (FDA) to regulate vitamins and other health products was defeated by a coalition of conservative and some liberal legislators with the support of a variety of alternative health care oriented organizations. All of this is occurring while the National Institutes of Health (NIH) has established the Office of Alternative Medicine (OAM), which has been the target of ridicule by some members of the medical establishment.[6] Nevertheless, its budget has increased from two million dollars when it first started to fifty million dollars in 1998 when it was upgraded from a program office to a full center (now called the National Center for Complementary and Alternative Medicine).

According to some this explosion of interest in non-allopathic forms of health care is in part rooted in a perception that various chronic and degenerative diseases ranging from severe allergies to AIDS to cancer have eluded successful conventional medical treatment. Ivan Illich's classic critique of medicine, *Medical Nemesis,* goes much farther in claiming that improvements in the health and well-being of modern societies is not the result of conventional medicine and its reliance on drugs and surgery. In fact, according to Illich, increases in longevity have occurred in spite of biomedicine, primarily as a result of improvements in nutrition, sanitation, and economic and technological advances.[7] Since Illich's work, other critiques of biomedicine have pointed to problems of unnecessary surgery, a rise of doctor-induced illness (iatrogenesis), and the overuse of antibiotics drugs, producing new strains of drug-resistant pathogens.[8] A recent study published in the *Journal of the American Medical Association* estimated that 106,000 hospital patients die and 2.2 million are injured each year by adverse reactions to prescription drugs, even if properly prescribed. Another study found that 6.5 percent of patients at two teaching hospitals in Boston had been injured by their medicines and one-third of these cases involved mistakes. This study became the basis for a front-page article in the *New York Times.*[9]

Until the last fifteen or twenty years it had been widely believed that acute infectious illnesses that terrified Western industrialized societies from cholera to tuberculosis to polio have been contained or cured through the use of antibiotics, vaccines, and public health measures.[10] Instead, chronic diseases, ailments that may have an acute phase but typically last for many years and can be medically managed but rarely cured, have become dominant.[11] Yet, if we take a global perspective, it is now no longer quite so simple. The return of malaria, legionnaire's disease, toxic shock, tuberculosis, the Ebola virus, and most significantly AIDS shows that infectious diseases are still with us, although most of these infectious diseases can be treated and managed.[12]

Nevertheless, in the more developed nations of the world, it is still largely accurate to talk about the rise of chronic disease, especially the "autoimmune disorders" such as asthma, rheumatoid arthritis, lupus, MS, and Crohn's disease.[13] The success as well of biomedicine (arguably) means that more patients with heart disease and cancer can survive for long periods. While rates of heart disease have just begun to decline, there is no evidence that the multibillion dollar war against cancer has achieved any but the most modest of successes. Indeed, it is estimated that one out of every three Americans will be afflicted with cancer in their lifetime.[14] These chronic and degenerative diseases have been resistant to the "magic bullet" approach of biomedicine. Even in the case of AIDS where a virus and mode of transmission have been identified, a cure is not in sight. In the case of other chronic diseases, there is a growing recognition that there are multiple factors, many of them environmental and social, that must be taken into account in understanding disease etiology.

In addition to these larger social and environmental factors, chronic disease foregrounds what Aronowitz calls "the problem of idiosyncrasy," what individuals bring to disease by virtue of their unique experience. Why, for example, does one HIV positive patient remain AIDS free for twenty years while another succumbs to the disease within a few months? Why do some patients with severe asthma do well with steroid inhalers while others fail to improve despite the treatment? What about those patients whose suffering does not have a name, or in other words does not lend itself to medicalization, until recently patients with "Chronic Fatigue Syndrome"? The inability to fully resolve the problem of idiosyncrasy is why historians of medicine have discovered a tension within biomedicine between those who adopt the now dominant reductionist project, which seeks to link every disease to a pathogen and a gene, and, on the other hand, the more holistic approach within biomedicine, represented by an earlier tradition of "psychosomatic medicine," the more recent risk factor approach to disease and the type A explanation for heart disease (linking heart disease to certain personality types and lifestyle patterns). In other words holistic and reductionist understandings of disease have coexisted even within biomedicine, although holistic views have been marginalized.[15]

Chronic illness often oscillates between periods when symptoms worsen and other periods of remission, when the ill person can function in a more or less normal fashion. It is quite common for patients with problems such as chronic back pain, arthritis, asthma, and Crohn's disease to see a variety of doctors, to experiment with a wide range of treatments and to see alternative practitioners.[16] The fact that these and other chronic illnesses can only be managed by conventional medicine (if that) and not cured means that people with these illnesses never feel entirely satisfied with the treatments they receive at the doctor's office.[17] Moreover, the persistence of chronic illness means that its effects will seep beyond the body into the person's relationships and self-identity. There is evidence that damage to the self and to a person's social networks can loop back into the experience of illness.[18] It is not surprising under these circumstances that there is increased interest in alternative health, in part because it offers a range of treatments that conventional medicine does not offer but also because of the emphasis in alternative health on healing as a change in how one lives as well as a change in the body. In short, the "epidemiological transition" from acute infectious diseases to chronic disease may be one of a number of factors explaining the growing challenge to biomedical hegemony.

This challenge to biomedical hegemony has other sources as well. Clearly, there are larger changes in American culture that have produced a climate or sensibility conducive to challenging medical authority. Alternative health's emphasis on patient empowerment is consistent with the larger critique of professional expertise and the medicalization of suffering in the feminist, hospice, and self-help movements.[19] Anyone taking a childbirth class in a major hospital will be exposed to these ideas in the form of Lamaze classes. In a subdued manner, women are encouraged to trust their bodies, rely on the wisdom of their mothers and grandmothers, and view childbirth as a natural process and not pathology. They and their partners learn various breathing exercises that the instructors hope will reduce the need for medical intervention. The best-selling *Our Bodies, Ourselves* is a manual of self-care and a critique of medicalization. The opening chapter in the latest edition is entitled, "Taking Care of Ourselves."[20]

In addition to this cultural emphasis on self-care, the spiritual renewal of the past forty years is another cultural resource that has encouraged a challenge to medical authority. Only here the point is not the reappropriation of skills monopolized by experts but the search for meaning. What McLoughlin calls "the fourth Great Awakening,"[21] beginning in the 1960s, challenged religious and scientific authority by reintroducing elements of Eastern and Native American spirituality, seeking a sense of God's immanence in the world through various experiences of mysticism and intimate forms of community ("communitas").[22] This yearning for connection to nature and the wider universe is a central feature of much of alternative health. Evangelical Christianity also experienced a rebirth during this period and though its political implications depart from the radicalism of the counterculture, born-again Christians sought a more intimate and emotional connection with God, in contrast to the formality and emphasis on God's transcendence in mainline Protestant denominations. In short, the movements that emerged from the "fourth Great Awakening" sought to reintegrate everyday life with larger horizons of meaning and establish new connections with the past and with diverse traditions.

To summarize, there are a number of factors contributing to the challenge to the hegemony of biomedicine. First, there is the changing nature of disease and the stubborn persistence of old forms of infectious disease that are becoming more difficult to manage. Second, cultural mutations rooted in the sixties provide pressure to reembed disease in frameworks of meaning and significance, that is, to respiritualize disease and loosen the grip of mechanistic models. Third, the resistance to authority that swept over the culture during this period also challenged medical authority and its monopoly over the definition and treatment of disease. The growing prominence of alternative health can be traced to this concatenation of changes.

What is Alternative Health?

How should alternative health be conceptualized? There are significant differences among the many approaches that are loosely labeled under the umbrella term *alternative health*. Some forms of alternative medicine emphasize the spiritual, psychological, and attitudinal bases for disease and healing. Attitudinal healing, past life regression, various forms of meditation, reiki, Christian Science, all point to a person's attitudes or spiritual condition as a central source of disease and the primary path to healing. Some spiritually oriented approaches claim that diseases are chosen by people as a way of experiencing and working out existential problems. On the other hand, approaches such as naturopathy, homeopathy, Ayurvedic medicine, and oxygen therapies, while recognizing psychological and spiritual dimensions, emphasize physical interventions such as the ingesting of herbs, drinking hydrogen peroxide, eating organic food, administering infusions of vitamin C, and taking homeopathic amounts (very low levels) of toxic material to stimulate the immune system. In addition, some forms of alternative medicine tend toward monocausal explanations of disease and their cure—oxidation approaches—while other approaches are more catholic in their understanding of disease and their remedies. In all these orientations the background intellectual traditions they draw upon vary widely and at times may conflict. For example, some approaches attempt to ground alternative health practices in biblical teachings and principles while others draw upon eastern religious and healing traditions and still others on Western metaphysical traditions.

The conflicts within alternative health do not just refer to disparate understandings of the field but extend also to the appropriate relationship to biomedicine and its associated institutions and to scientific approaches to health care claims. Schools of naturopathy offer a standard array of courses, similar to what one might find at a medical school, although the curriculum also includes courses in nutrition, botanical medicine, and Ayurvedic medicine. In contrast, training for other health care practitioners de-emphasizes science and focuses on either spiritual or exotic healing strategies and courses. For the School of Holistic Theology, alternative health is more akin to steps in the process of spiritual understanding than a scientific enterprise. They also oppose accreditation and therefore the official recognition and legitimation of their movement. Some alternative practitioners we talked to would like very much to see some of their claims subjected to standard scientifically controlled double blind studies, which they cannot conduct because of the enormous expense involved. On the other hand, more spiritually oriented practitioners and other more militant sectors oppose any contact with biomedicine and view standard scientific modes of verification as deficient because one cannot quantify and capture all the variables involved in true healing.

In light of these differences, should the category of "alternative health" still be used? Does its use obscure more than it illuminates? Is there nothing that unites these diverse approaches other than their difference from the dominant system of biomedicine? Moreover, does this negative definition obscure the fact that biomedicine is not monolithic and, as was discussed earlier, has a holistic dimension? In the end we are convinced, along with many others, that the term must be used, although with some caution not to reify it, treating "it" as a unified rather than diverse and contradictory phenomenon. It is the term most widely used today by health activists and professionals, government officials, and others even though we are also seeing a new term, "complementary and alternative medicine," used in some contexts. Across Europe as well, "alternative health" or "alternative medicine" is the most widely used characterization.[23] Moreover, with the reemergence of alternative health, we now find growing connections between various alternative health professions and among various groups. Alternative health participants share a collective identity, a sense of "we," and see themselves as members of a common community and movement. There is also some organizational coherence as diverse segments of the community form alliances with one another in common organizations in order to advance their collective interests. This reflects not only the need to unite against a common opponent but the development of a critique of biomedicine that is quite similar across the many branches of alternative health. At least part of the reason for the emergence of this collective identity may be that the medical establishment, since the 1970s, has largely chosen to characterize various groups of non-allopathic professionals under the generic term *alternative* rather than referring to a specific modality (such as acupuncture or chiropractic). This was, as Cant and Sharma argue, a response to the perception of a new challenge, the reemergence of alternative health.[24] In a more positive sense, there is also a common philosophy that underlies the varieties of alternative modalities and settings within which alternative practitioners work. Despite the real differences in the set of protocols they are committed to, what tradition they have been trained in, and the institutional setting in which they work, the practitioners and activists we interviewed can provide a coherent approach to health and illness.[25]

At the core of alternative health is a commitment to an ecological conception of the body, in which biochemical processes, emotional states, beliefs, lifestyle practices (especially nutrition), and spiritual phenomena are thought to be interconnected. While we will argue that this holism is incomplete and often fails to appreciate the social and class dimensions of illness, everyone in the alternative health community espouses the principle. A wide range of alternative healing systems posit an interconnected world, in which biological states are expressions of interactions with wider systems. Disease is not so much an attack by an outside agent but a disruption of an inherent balance between body, self, spirit, and wider environment. According to one writer,

> Good health—in its broadest sense—occurs when we live in harmony with our selves and our environment, maintaining a balance in the face of changes, growing with challenges, and developing our innate healing powers. In essence, to be healthy is to be integrated and whole.[26]

Beyond this emphasis on holism, there is also a commitment to low-tech care, individualized treatment regimes (treating the person not the symptom), in which the patient's experiences, intuitions, and perceptions of his or her illness are an important part of diagnosis and treatment. To the extent to which this principle fully informs practice, alternative health relentlessly opposes the "medicalization" of a patient's distress. A person's symptoms—lower back pain, allergies, and intestinal pain—are related to larger elements of the person's life. More often than not, the practitioner refrains from using a diagnostic category to characterize the symptoms, in part because of the belief that this will only trap the person in the "sick role" and at the same time limit the practitioner's effort to uncover wider connections.[27]

There is also an emphasis on the self-healing capacities of the body. Here, all varieties of alternative health posit some fundamental state of balance between the person and nature that allows for healing. For many in alternative medicine, this idea is expressed through the modern scientific language of psychoneuroimmunology, the claim, which is now receiving serious scientific attention, that there is a strong relationship between one's emotional state and the healing capacities of the body and that activating this internal healing capacity through inducing certain emotions or states of mind can have a healing effect.[28] For others, recourse is made to categories that come from traditional healing systems—the *qi* of Chinese medicine, or the "vital breath" of Ayurvedic medicine. Here, vitalism replaces the mechanistic view of biomedicine. There is a flow of life or energy that connects the person to the wider universe. It follows that healing is more a function of what the person does to regain a lost state of balance, or to "activate the immune system," than it is the function of the expert to cure a diseased body.

This emphasis on the self-healing capacities of the body implies a commitment to something more than the absence of disease—to "wellness" or some positive conception of health. We will discuss this positive conception of health in more detail in chapter 4, in terms of our notion of alternative health's "classical aesthetic project." In some respects this can be understood as a greater emphasis on preventive medicine but it is important here not to confuse this term with the way it is commonly used in biomedicine. Prevention, in alternative medicine, refers to the totality of how one lives one's life. The food we eat, our posture and how we hold our bodies, the quality of our relationships, the pace and stress of our work, the state of our "soul" are all part of the process of staying healthy. Prevention, here, is more than coming in for the yearly medical checkup.

Self-healing and a positive conception of health require a different model of expertise than the dominant one in biomedicine. There is a desire in alternative medicine to narrow the power imbalances between practitioner and patient. It is common in alternative health to refer to patients as "partners" in the healing process. Usually this means that patients are expected to be active in suggesting treatments, asking questions, looking up the latest information on the Internet, and in general educating themselves about their illnesses. The notion of partnership also refers to the expectation, especially for serious illnesses, that patients will engage in "self-care," daily healing regimes that are more or less tailored to the specific needs of each person. The expert may help the patient in devising her regime but ultimately it is up to the person to make the daily adjustments and changes and of course to do the work of shopping, juicing, cooking and preparing, fasting and cleansing that is an integral part of this process of self-care. Finally, patients in alternative health are "partners" with their practitioners because healing is thought to involve an examination of how the person lives her life—her thought patterns, eating habits, relationships, and lifestyle. Getting healthy often involves a fundamental reexamination of all these things. The practitioner can point the way but only the ill person can accomplish this.

In other words, the ecological view of the body is embedded in an ongoing practice. In contrast to the passive role of the patient in allopathic medicine, the patient plays an active role in her recovery and maintenance of health. This involves a greater reciprocity between health provider and patient and may involve forms of self-administered care. Patients are no longer recipients of expertise and therapies, monopolized by the provider. In this way persons are thought to regain "responsibility for their health." Patients actively administer protocols in individualized ways depending on the context and the health problem. This is possible because alternative medicine does not depend on complex technological interventions, allowing anyone with reasonable skill to engage in self-care.

Finally, alternative medicine draws upon traditional practices and beliefs, many of which are not based on the dominant model of scientific testing. Instead, the apparent effectiveness of these treatments is attributed to their use over long periods of time. Protocols are legitimated by virtue of their endurance, an evocation of the authority of tradition. The reliance on the wisdom of the past does not mean that treatments are employed uncritically or without attention to whether or not they work for particular patients. Indeed, even traditional healing systems are not oblivious to the efficacy of their healing practices. Instead, at least part of the attractiveness of alternative health is that it relies on a scarce commodity in the modern world, the "wisdom" of the past, in coping with one of life's fundamental exigencies.

Lowenberg calls this understanding of health and illness the "new model of health care." This model is consistent with the philosophy just outlined and has the following constituents: illness as imbalance or "dis-ease"; treating the cause of the disease not symptoms; illness as opportunity for self-growth and self-discovery; individual responsibility for health; practitioners as educators, consultants, facilitators; the practitioner mobilizing the innate healing capacities of the body; the practitioner and physical setting is to be warm, caring, and encouraging the patient to feel highly valued; an egalitarian relationship between practitioner and patient (in fact, most practitioners do not call the people they work on patients); and finally, the practitioner as a role model, embodying the health he is trying to stimulate in the patient.[29] While we use the term *alternative health* throughout this book, we also use the term *complementary medicine* to refer to the use of non-allopathic approaches to healing in a medical setting, and we use the term *holistic* to refer to one way in which alternative health practices are understood.

One way of illustrating the contrast between biomedicine and alternative medicine is through a review of strategies for treating cancer as well as "candidiasis," an overgrowth of yeast in the intestinal system. There is much debate among medical researchers, and a lack of consensus about the etiology of the many forms of cancer. While diagnosis remains technologically sophisticated, treatments center around the use of radiation, surgery, and chemotherapy. Treatment has had some success, but death rates for the major killers such as lung, colon, and breast cancer have remained high over many decades. According to one study only 2 to 3 percent of all cancer patients diagnosed each year are cured using chemotherapy, radiation, or surgery (or some combination).[30] Underlying these older and emerging treatment regimes is a focus on disease isolatable to a particular organ or process in the body even though treatments are nonspecific in their effects, killing both healthy and cancerous cells. Interventions such as chemotherapy are designed to attack a particular form of cancer as it manifests itself in a specific location.

On the other hand, alternative health practitioners, whether located in an alternative cancer clinic or elsewhere, focus on enhancing the body's immune system through dietary regimes (such as macrobiotics and the supersaturation of the body through the juicing of organic fruits and vegetables), megavitamin therapy, oxidation therapy, lifestyle changes, psychological and spiritual approaches such as guided imagery and meditation.[31] While there are differences in emphasis among practitioners of these various therapies, all agree that the cancer is not in the tumor but in the breakdown of the harmony and balance of the body. Treatment, therefore, must not be limited to the removal of tumors but to general bodily rejuvenation and reestablishing a proper balance between the person and the wider world.

Candidiasis, according to alternative health practitioners, is a chronic problem that can be either specific to the intestines or can be systemic, causing generalized problems in the body ranging from allergies to sleep disorders to malabsorption of food. Conventional treatment attempts to kill the yeast through drug specific intervention such as the use of Nistantin and Nizoral, among others. In contrast, alternative health practitioners employ more holistic protocols. Many practitioners will recommend an alteration of diet that includes elimination of sugar and simple carbohydrates and an emphasis upon vegetables, complex carbohydrates, and protein in proper combinations. Also, what is needed, in the alternative view, is the repopulation of the intestinal track with favorable flora that help to eliminate the yeast overgrowth. Supplements such as garlic and grapefruit seed extract may be also be recommended. In one case the object is to eliminate the pathogen while in the other the object is to rebuild the immune system so that the body itself can restore the proper balance of bacteria in the intestinal track. As we will discuss later, the alternative health protocols recommended to eliminate candidiasis do not end when the symptoms are longer present. Instead, they become incorporated into an ongoing practice that changes the person's life.

As we will discuss later, biomedicine is particularly interested in the diagnoses of disease and it is this process that most interests physicians.

After all, diagnosis provides puzzles, for which biomedicine has a wide range of tools with a high degree of technological sophistication. But, by and large, treatment is less refined. There are limited tools here, in the biomedical arsenal. Antibiotics and drugs are the principal forms of bio-medical intervention but according to recent studies there is little under-standing of why drugs work when they do and even less understanding of interaction effects between drugs when they are prescribed. Surgery is the other major intervention but here too recent studies show that this therapeutic tool is often overused and many forms of surgery are of questionable value (surgery for back pain).

On the other hand, alternative health is not particularly interested in the etiology of disease, identifying a precise biological mechanism responsible for an underlying disorder. Nor is there much interest in labeling an illness with a specific disease category. As mentioned earlier, to do so would be to risk trapping the person in a passive role rather than encouraging responsibility for their recovery. Moreover, waiting until someone has a "disease" before offering them care is also outside the framework of alternative health. A person may be "out of balance," have "trigger points," or just be out of energy and exhausted without having a legitimate disease. Still, a practitioner will try to devise, with the person's input, a treatment regime. In other words, most of the effort of the practitioner is dedicated to treatment. Treatment, in alternative health, can range from psychological and spir-itual approaches, to nutritional regimes, to the use of herbs and home-opathic remedies. In other words, treatment strategies are not symptom specific since the effort is to treat the whole person and as a result precise diagnosis is not as compelling. Typically, a wide range of treat-ments is pragmatically employed depending on the idiosyncratic aspects of the individual's illness. Self-care also requires a fine-tuning of treatment by the patient herself so that it meets her specific needs. So, alternative practitioners employ a two-track methodology. One the one hand, they treat the whole person through a range of protocols that does not require a precise diagnosis. On the other hand, they will fine-tune element of a variety of protocols to meet the specific needs of the patient.

While it's important to clarify differences between alternative health and biomedicine, the notion of some in alternative health that it is a dis-tinctively new paradigm as well as its characterization of biomedicine should not be accepted uncritically. Biomedicine is not hostile to all therapies considered "alternative" and periodically holistic challenges to biomedical orthodoxy arise from within the dominant paradigm. There seems to be some divergence between the official stance of biomedicine and the actual practice of many physicians who use some alternative therapies in their practices.[32] There are, as some argue, multiple forms of knowledge within biomedicine, "analytic knowledge," which revolves around the clinical encounter of doctor and patient, as well as the more dominant experimental and "techno-science" forms of knowledge. The emphasis in clinical medicine is on what works with particular patients, understanding disease in the specific biographical context of the patient, even if this form of knowledge in not dominant in biomedicine.[33] Moreover, as we will see throughout the book, the claim of many activists that alternative health is entirely distinct from biomedicine may obscure orientations that it shares with biomedicine and that blind both to a deeper critique of the health care system.

The Study of Alternative Health

There have been a number of academic studies of alternative health care practices. Earlier studies have marginalized alternative medicine through the use of an evolutionary paradigm that saw alternative medicine as a cultural curiosity, a survival from simpler social formations. In this perspective, alternative medicine is a fossil, which illustrates a process of incomplete modernization. Practices that some call "folk medicine" become in this view childish and prerational, held by the unsophisticated and those with low social status.[34] Functionalist and psychological theories have seen alternative medicine as a response to conditions under which people have lost control of their lives. These practices function to relieve anxiety and stress, restoring a prior balance in relation to the person's environment. These health practices may also have socially integrative consequences, bringing the patient together with family members and others in the community. But functionalist explanations that explain the consequences of alternative medicine in terms of the needs of larger structures don't take seriously the claims of actors. In other words, folk medicine is explained away by appealing to a reified view of society as having needs and purposes, independent of actors. Biomedicine is assumed to embody truthful accounts of the world and how it operates. Yet the same functionalist arguments can equally explain the existence of allopathic medicine—with the same unsatisfactory result.[35]

While research on alternative health within the sociology of medicine lacks this clear and overt bias, much of it examines alternative health from the vantage point of biomedicine. It assumes that alternative health can be understood as a marginal medical practice focusing on professionalization of alternative health therapies or how patients make decisions about treatment.[36] The key questions explored within the sociology of medicine revolve around explaining why patients choose alternative practitioners and how they compare with patients of conventional M.D.s, describing how alternative clinics operate and exploring the relationship between alternative health practitioners and the dominant healthcare system. Rarely is alternative health placed within the context of larger social and cultural change.[37]

Lowenberg's study is one of the most detailed treatments of the interaction between alternative and allopathic medicine. Lowenberg explores a new model of the patient, which emerges out of alternative/holistic medicine. This new model alters the traditional relationship between patient and doctor by emphasizing new values and responsibilities. For example, patients in the holistic model are required to "take responsibility for their health," which may mean assuming blame for their illness and doing the work required to overcome it. This new model, Lowenberg argues, rejects the "sick role model" formulated by Talcott Parsons. The sick role model posits a set of rights and obligations that are incorporated in the role of the ill person in modern societies. In return for following medical authority and the protocols they establish (which includes the effort to get well), the sick person receives an exemption from work and from responsibility for the cause of the illness.

The core of Lowenberg's book is an examination of a family clinic where allopathic and holistic approaches to health care are combined. Practitioners prescribe drugs and other conventional modalities along with holistic treatments such as acupuncture, biofeedback and stress reduction, colon therapy and nutritional counseling. Lowenberg's chief question is how contradictions in the holistic model are worked out in practice. One contradiction within the holistic model is the assumption of patient responsibility for illness, which may subvert the self-understanding of the practitioner as caring and compassionate. Another contradiction is the attempt to graft onto the holistic model biomedical practices that increase the authority of the doctor as having authoritative expertise and who can unilaterally devise a cure.[38] Overall, Lowenberg argues that the allopathic model of medical expertise in relation to the patient is compromised but not overturned in this setting. Practitioners maintain a caring, compassionate stance while continuing to relieve patients of responsibility for their illness and recovery, thus combining elements of allopathic and holistic models.

The most recent work within the sociology of medicine framework presents a critical sociological treatment of alternative medicine's relationship to biomedicine, the state, and consumers. These works conceptualize the current challenges to biomedicine as a "reemergence of medical pluralism." Hans Baer's recent work provides a critical and historical analysis of "medical pluralism," the shifting relations between biomedicine and other "medical subsystems."[39] He provides a detailed historical treatment of the wide range of alternative systems, their degree of professionalization and the extent to which they challenge the hegemony of biomedicine. Baer's placement of this history in the context of the changing political economy of American capitalism also provides a macro perspective that has thus far been missing in the literature.

Despite this valuable effort to place alternative health systems in a larger political-economic perspective and to understand alternative medicine's shifting interaction with the state, consumers, and biomedicine, alternative health systems are largely treated as embryonic or partially developed professions who are in a subordinate position in a larger system of medical pluralism. While we have found much of value in this work, what is missing is a focus on the lifeworld of patients and health activists, the way alternative health networks transform the identities of patients and the larger political implications of these changes. As we will discuss later, alternative health exists on a variety of levels of power, from the web of connections and associations that exist in everyday life to the level of organization and interest group politics and the level of political elites. What is most significant about alternative health, and the source of its creativity can be found in this first level, the lifeworld. In other words, the "new medical pluralism" perspective still confines alternative health to the institutional sphere of health, and to the levels of organization and elite decision-making processes.

Other approaches view alternative forms of healing as coherent belief systems that have to be grasped in terms of the language internal to them. Here the point is not to judge the truth-value of these systems but to make an effort to reconstruct the actors' interpretation of the world in terms of the standards embedded in its larger cultural contexts. One strategy in reconstructing the actors' interpretation of the world is through the analysis of cultural texts and their meaning. The researcher examines the meanings people construct about their illness and recovery experiences. For example, O'Connor studied a Hmong man who was diagnosed with severe liver disease. After a stay in the hospital, which included intravenous feeding, he was told that he needed a liver transplant. But for the Hmong, the liver is the seat of the soul and the center of the human personality. Healing for the Hmong is not accomplished through physical interventions, but through shamanic practices, which help to restore a balance between invisible fluids and energies. In addition, intravenous feeding meant that his stable diet of rice was unavailable, which the Hmong believes is an essential part of adequate nourishment. An acceptable medical treatment could only occur after doctors made their own interventions compatible with Hmong beliefs. For example, the patient was fed with intravenous rice water and liver transplant surgery was canceled in favor of protocols compatible with the patient's world view.[40]

Another variant of this approach is the use of narration to explore the cultural world of patients. The researcher constructs a structural model identifying the common property of the stories people tell about their illnesses and recovery. For Arthur Frank, the suffering that accompanies illness creates a need in the self for meaning through narration. Frank develops a typology of illness narratives from restitution stories, which seek through medical treatment to restore a prior condition of health, to chaos stories, which construct a spiral of unmanageable threats that engulf and overwhelm the person, to quest narratives, which find in illness opportunities for learning and integration of the self at higher levels of meaning. Frank argues that in the postmodern era there is a proliferation of self-constructed stories assembled from the wreckage caused by the rationalizing pressures of modernity. While all these stories have different textures, they are all shaped by a sense of "embodied paranoia." Institutions that are designed to help people appear as instruments of torture and threats to bodily integrity (chemotherapy, radiation, and medical life-support technologies).[41] In Scarry's words, these practices are "deworlding." They create levels of pain that make it impossible for people to establish normal connections with themselves and the world around them. Radical pain is privatizing.[42] What is interesting about Frank's analysis is that it raises an issue that we take up in the course of this work—the relationship among tradition, meaning, and autonomy in connection to health and illness.

In her ethnography McGuire also tries to sympathetically grasp the attraction of alternative health to sectors of the American middle class. She provides evidence and the beginning of an explanation for why "nonmedical healing" flourishes among an educated group whose sympathies one might assume would be more wedded to the biomedical model. For McGuire, nonmedical healing expresses opposition to "the rationalization of the body and emotions in contemporary society." Rationalization is understood in a Weberian sense as the absorption of actors into instrumental relationships in which their emotional and spiritual dimensions are erased. The link between a person's body and his self-identity is severed in conventional medicine through an expropriation of health by the dominant allopathic system. Overall, McGuire's work is valuable in describing the attachment of sectors of the middle class to a broader conception of healing than the biomedical model. But the institutional and cultural sources of this commitment are incompletely and only intermittently explored.[43]

There are also those who approach health and illness within a postmodern framework. Other approaches share with postmodernism a concern with questions of power that are implicated in doctor-patient relationships and how patients have tried to contest medical expertise. But postmodernism pushes the analysis one step farther. The very idea of expertise and the discourses that legitimate it becomes another exercise of power, which can claim no privileged status. The focus here is on strategies of evasion and resistance to experts and their medical discourse. These strategies of resistance can be described but not normatively grounded.

Nicolaus Fox, in his study of patients who are being subjected to postsurgical medical rounds, explores the way doctor-patient relationships inscribe a dominant discourse and stabilize a power relationship, which is then evaded in subtle and microscopic ways by patients. For example, subtleties of language and inflection are examined as instances of an ongoing power struggle in which doctors employ biomedical discourse in order to create a particular subjectivity and inscribe this onto bodies through medical practices.[44]

According to Honneth, postmodernism is a project that pursues the intensification of experiences independent of normative constraints.[45] The goal is simply more experience. This can take any form but in postmodernist texts there is a partiality for the self-experimentation of those on the margins and as a result stigmatized. In the case of illness this means a partiality for those who resist the allopathic model. Modernist medicine is rejected because its hegemonic discourse, based on a narrative of progress, marginalizes all other orientations. Where this leads us in terms of an alternative vision of health is unclear. Postmodernism could not frontally endorse any version of alternative health without violating its own premises. The notion that there is a conception and a practice of health that is closer to the truth than others violates the postmodern injunction against foundationalism and its connection to the metanarrative of progress. The relationship, therefore, of postmodernism to alternative health is unclear.

While the relationship between postmodernism and alternative health remains undeveloped and undefined, this is not the case (according to some scholars) with the fitness and wellness movements. Barry Glassner argues that fitness activities have little connection to earlier "modernist" projects of social regeneration—improving personal health as a path to national revitalization. Instead, the object is to transform the self—"to disengage the body rather than put them to the service of building a better America."[46] Second, fitness is not based on a linear view of progress or individual development. Fitness activities promise an escape from the "narrative of aging." Third, fitness activities "fragment bodies." Different body parts can be "worked" with different machines, and images of bodies no longer are structured around the old modernist polarities of inside-outside, male-female, and work-leisure. Finally, fitness activities are a pastiche, "perpetually reconstructed of pieces and colorations added on and then discarded." These pieces are not originals but are themselves images or "simulacra."[47]

This analysis of fitness as a postmodern activity falls far short of our earlier description of postmodernism and its underlying cultural commitments. For one thing, fitness is not a movement on the margins. People are not stigmatized who engage in it. On the contrary, dominant institutions positively encourage it, if not compel it and the media celebrates it in a panorama of image. Furthermore, intensification is anemic compared to the Nietzchean inspired concept of intoxication and its associations with madness, danger, and transgression of normal boundaries.

To be sure, this study of fitness breaks out of the narrow institutional model that characterizes some of the alternative health literature. Fitness is examined in terms of larger social and political changes, for example, periods of national regeneration, postmodernism, and changing consumer preferences. While alternative health is at times confused with the "fitness movement" we see fitness as a clearly distinct phenomenon, even if it embodies a weak form of the postmodern sensibility. In contrast, we are interested in alternative health's relationship to social change from the point of view of its capacity to resist dominant institutions and practices and to serve as a basis for their transformation. We also will embed our treatment of alternative health in the context of larger institutional dynamics.

All of these more sympathetic studies of alternative health tend to confine themselves to the terrain of health as an institutional sphere or stay on the level of the self and its interactions with medical experts. No doubt these approaches possess considerable value but we want to press the analysis of alternative health in several new directions, beyond the institutional sphere of health and the tribulations of the self. A critical theory of society is either omitted or only indirectly suggested in the work we have summarized. A critical theory of society examines the "total social process" as it is implicated in the contradictions of specific social practices.[48] Critical theories also thematize the way institutions repress human subjects as well as pointing to sources of resistance and transformation.[49]

We want to locate, in this spirit, alternative health in connection with the institutional and cultural dynamics of modern state-managed capitalist systems. The principal feature of these systems is the growing bureaucratization and commodification of more and more aspects of social life. These processes work their way through the health care system and reach into the lives of patients. Alternative health, as we will argue, occupies a contradictory position in relation to this process, being at one and the same time complementary and source of resistance to it. In existing state capitalist systems, traditional sources of resistance and change—class conflict—have weakened as a result of the growth of the welfare state and the right of workers to bargain for a share of it. At the same time, new forms of conflict have emerged outside of the economic system, which new social movement theorists have tried to conceptualize. Unstudied in this respect is alternative health as an expression of new forms of conflict, which have transformative potential.

While the use of a social movements perspective means that we do not focus on distinct therapies and their efforts to professionalize or on the way individual patients make decisions about treatment, this view does have the advantage of emphasizing the politics of alternative health; the extent to which involvement in this community politicizes participants and the relationship between alternative health and other movements. Despite the organization of alternative health into distinct therapies, many of which have their own professional associations, in practice most practitioners use a range of alternative therapies, and the gap in expertise between practitioner and the committed patient is not great. As we will argue later, a focus on the individual patient or on professionalization neglects the significance of alternative health as a "cultural laboratory," where information is shared, identities are transformed, and new values emerge. A social movements perspective can evaluate whether alternative health is part of a larger project of social change and whether it is more than a niche in the health care market.

Within the context of alternative health as a social movement, we are also concerned with alternative health as a source of personal identity, the appropriation of meaning and the ways in which alternative health regimes allow people to "care for the self"—all of which have an internal relationship with the capacities of actors to commit themselves to wider social changes. In this analysis we draw on the works of Walter Benjamin, Michel Foucault, Charles Taylor, and Alberto Melucci in order to comprehend the interaction between the self and alternative health networks.

Loss of Tradition and Autonomy

Alternative health is implicated in the problems of tradition and the transmissibility of the past. Here we will use the work of Walter Benjamin, Max Weber, and the more recent insights of new social movement theory to illuminate how alternative health is a complex response to the loss of meaning or (what amounts to the same thing) the collapse of tradition in modern societies.

Various branches of alternative medicine seek to appropriate and sustain health practices and traditions that in some cases go back thousands of years. In appropriating healing traditions, alternative health participants seek to reestablish a connection with past generations. In this way the "circle of life" is partially renewed at the level of care for the body.[50] These traditions; Chinese medicine, Ayurvedic medicine, macrobiotics, Native American and other indigenous healing traditions, for example, have been marginalized by the dominance of biomedicine. Biomedicine is an application of specialized research engaged in by experts with institutional support from the state and universities. This research is detached from the self-understandings and conversations of people in everyday life. Moreover, biomedicine's interventions do not require an understanding of the patient's subjective world, competencies, and the roots that give it meaning. As a result, the way we care for our physical well-being has become detached from the larger "lifeworld" and its continuities with the past. In other words, expertise becomes increasingly detached from the self-understandings of actors in everyday life. In this sense, the recovery of alternative health care practices is implicated in this larger crisis concerning the past and its formative influence.

Alternative health groups seek to defend the validity of traditional health care practices and the "form of life" that is embedded in them. This form of life, though, is peculiar. It does not mean an actual existing organic community threatened by modernization. Instead, what is threatened is an "imagined community" that traces its roots back to diverse practices of many traditions. The term *imagined community* or what Hobsbawm calls "invented traditions" suggests an invented connection to the past constructed for political purposes.[51] For example, certain myths and rituals connected to the British monarchy were created in order to legitimate existing power relations. But, we argue, this political use of the past does not exhaust the ways in which people gain access to tradition in modern societies. Instead, we claim that in alternative health traditions are transmitted and maintained through the body and its travails. In other words, this contact with the past is not just an intellectual recovery described in books and newspapers or inscribed in state-sanctioned ceremonies but is instead rooted in experience. It was Proust who wrote that we gain access to the past by tasting tangible things, which contain memories in material form. So too, in alternative health the past offers itself up in the form of material things and the memories inscribed in them. The body and its care become the transmitter of the past in usable form.

An example can be found in any of the alternative health fairs that occur on a regular basis throughout the country. Indian music and ancient forms of drumming can be heard while various booths display Chinese herbal health remedies, acupuncture, Native American charms and amulets. All of this takes place in an environment where everyone is selling their wares much like merchants in a market. This is a good example of what Lowenberg calls the "translation of eastern philosophy into western terms of utilitarian individualism."[52] Here we find traditions selectively lifted from their original context and redeployed in a Western commercial setting. Continuities with the past here are imagined in the sense that they can be selectively displayed without having a shaping influence on everyday life. What is weakened here is the binding force of tradition, its capacity to obligate us. We reserve for future discussion the question of the significance of the past when it can no longer be drawn upon but merely displayed. This question is the same one that Walter Benjamin raised when he argued that meaning and happiness depends on the renewal of the semantic potentials embedded in tradition and asked whether that renewal is possible under the conditions of modern life.

In addition to the problem of the past and its transmissibility, we also explore the problem of autonomy in relation to the institution-alized provision of health care. Alternative health practices are one source of opposition to dominant institutions and a vehicle for their potential transformation. In other words, alternative health is impli-cated in another dimension of modernity that Max Weber emphasized, the loss of autonomy. Insofar as the world becomes rationalized, it becomes locked in bureaucratic forms of control and surveillance—the "iron cage of total administration."[53] In the same spirit Habermas argues that the lifeworld becomes colonized through the media of wealth and power. In other words, instead of people organizing them-selves through their own communicative efforts, people become linked behind their backs by administrative power and money. Alternative health, we argue, is a response to the colonization of the lifeworld. This response is enacted through the formation of "subaltern public spaces" where subjects and topics can be freely discussed by partici-pants, providing a space for innovation in health practices. Here alter-native health generates "space for more autonomous construction of group identity and political deliberation."

Food co-ops, alternative cancer groups, study groups, lectures, and alternative health organizations involve sharing information, formu-lating common values and principles, and deliberating about the impact of legislative proposals and government regulations. In this sense alternative health is not only about the continuation of imagined traditions but the creation of new modes of interaction and contes-tation. The exchange of alternative health information empowers people to develop competencies with respect to their health and illness and to act upon conditions that endanger them. Alternative health groups seek to reappropriate skills that modern institutions have removed from them, for example, knowledge of food production and preparation, and self-healing techniques. These subaltern public spaces are aimed at self-care (the freedom to supervise one's health) and insti-tutional contestation (challenging the state and it's regulatory and research functions in connection to the medical industrial complex). To be an unconventional health care practitioner is to face numerous obstacles that come from state regulatory agencies. These obstacles include the lack of state-supported funding for alternative health research, problems of licensing and official recognition, and in some cases criminalization of certain alternative health modalities.

We are conceptualizing alternative health as a social movement, rather than consumption choices and lifestyle decisions of individuals. This perspective allows us to explore alternative health's connections outside the sphere of health, to other social movements and subcultures. Our analysis will show that alternative health provides a cultural laboratory or site of experimentation from which social movements draw their energy, purpose, and orientation. At the same time, alternative health has implications for interest group struggles that shape state policies as well as the values and orientations of elite decision makers.

In summary, alternative health is an attempt to protect endangered ways of life through invented traditions and pursues new forms of life through spaces for dialogue and discussion as conditions for individual and collective action. These attempts to pursue both meaning and autonomy create problems and unintended consequences, which future chapters will explore. Do invented traditions really transmit the past in a morally binding way and therefore serve to orient actors in everyday life? Can subaltern health publics generate enough energy to challenge the medical-industrial complex and related institutions? Can alternative medicine fulfill its own potential in challenging biomedicine without going beyond its fixation on the individual and on the market? In other words, how far can alternative health proceed on the path from lifeworld to politics in its present form? The following chapters will explore these questions beginning with the origins and nature of biomedicine, its relationship to the lifeworld of patients and the nature of expertise in alternative health. If alternative health is in part a movement that seeks to reembed health and illness in the lifeworld of patients, then we need to begin by examining biomedicine's relationship to this process.

CHAPTER 2

Biomedicine and the Loss of Meaning

Biomedicine

Biomedicine and the more general process of modernization are riddled with paradoxes. On the one hand, modern medicine is a vehicle for the creation in society of greater health and well-being but, on the other hand, it has led to rising rates of doctor-created disease, which has been well documented. For example, a recent study demonstrates that approximately 106,000 people die of prescription drugs every year even when properly prescribed.[1] According to other studies 98,000 people die each year of improper medical interventions such as botched operations, improperly prescribed drugs, and other forms of negligence within hospitals.[2] In a larger sense medical progress is running up against its potential limits in the form of overuse of antibiotics and the appearance of drug resistant pathogens, spiraling health care costs, and medicine's inability to make headway against a range of chronic diseases from cancer to many autoimmune diseases despite momentary miracle claims to the contrary.

In addition, the prestige of medicine and its connection to the project of progress and enlightenment has its underside in the form of cultural impoverishment leading to a loss of meaning in the lifeworld. Major life transitions such as birth, illness, and death were once encoded in ritual and larger cultural horizons. These rituals and horizons fall apart as they become subject to medical analysis and intervention.[3] In this chapter we will explore the growing tension between progress and the achievements of biomedicine and its unintended impact on meaning in everyday life.

We use the term *biomedicine* here as opposed to Western or conventional medicine because biomedicine has achieved global dominance. It is misleading to think of it as only one of many healing systems and certainly not one that is geographically confined to Western societies. Biomedicine has displaced or at least marginalized many indigenous healing systems throughout the world. Moreover, the term *conventional* does not adequately emphasize biomedicine's scientific claims, and reductionist project. The term *scientific medicine* would be inappropriate because it implies that "science" is coterminous with biomedicine, rather than viewing biomedicine as one of a number of scientific approaches to medicine. Despite very real differences in its relationship to other healing systems and to the state in different countries, there is a good deal of cross-cultural consistency in the nature of biomedicine as a profession.

Biomedicine in America has its origins in the Cartesian world view in which body and mind are separated. The body is then construed to work according to mechanical principles independent of the will, spirituality, and purposes of the subject. In other words, the patients' subjective lifeworld remains external to medical diagnosis and treatment. This world view orients biomedicine and provides its principal justification. Biomedicine conceives of itself as an embodiment of scientific principles that serve as the primary source of its authority and legitimation. Biomedicine attempts to repair, replace, or revive processes in the body through surgery, immunizations, and, most importantly, the use of prescription drugs.[4]

Biomedicine was born in a field of conflict with competing approaches: homeopathy, botanical medicine, hydrotherapy, Christian Science, and a variety of spiritually oriented approaches which at least in part contested the Cartesian world view.[5] For example, the Thomsonians in the early and mid-nineteenth century believed that all disease had one cause, lack of sufficient heat in the body, and one cure—various herbal treatments and hot baths to generate heat and energy. The Thomsonian movement in the early nineteenth century was part of the larger Jacksonian wave of protest against "the system of regular medicine" and professionals of all sorts (ministers, lawyers, bankers). The movement aimed "to make every man his own physician." Around the same period of time Sylvester Graham, a Presbyterian minister, led a health movement against various forms of "overstimulation," excessive intake of alcohol, overstimulation of the sexual organs, and overeating. These excesses were in turn understood as a transgression against "God's laws." The solution, he argued, was to ensure that the stomach and intestinal system were supplied with a proper (and limited supply) of food, since this was the body's source of "vital power." He was the nineteenth century's most famous advocate of a vegetarian diet, placing special emphasis on ingesting bread made from coarse wheat flour rather than refined flour.

Homeopathy is based on the belief that disease could be cured through the application of very diluted dosages of substances similar to the disease. Unlike Thomsonianism and Grahamism, homeopathy did not begin as a popular movement but instead came from the ranks of the medical profession. Its founder, Samuel Christina Hahnenmann, a German physician, established the principle that "like is cured by like." Drugs should be prescribed that produce symptoms similar to the patient's. This principle was based on his view that disease is not an underlying condition causing symptoms but instead that there are only the patient's symptoms. "A disease in its whole range is represented only by the complex of morbid symptoms . . ." In other words, homeopathy paid close attention to the patient's accounts of her illness and remedies were tailored to the specifics of the patient's condition.

The second principle of homeopathy is that patients receive the greatest therapeutic benefit when dosages are small ("the doctrine of infinitesimals"). Only the smallest dosage is needed to produce a dynamic effect, while larger dosages only damage the body's ability to overcome the disease. The homeopathic dose, they argued, produced a weaker and more easily treated version of the disease that the patient's body could easily overcome. Finally, homeopathy like many other nineteenth-century healing systems asserted that true healing tapped into a "vital spirit" that could stimulate the body's capacity to heal itself. The popularity of homeopathy with physicians and the general public is in large part responsible for the formation by regular physicians of the American Medical Association (AMA), in order to advance their interests.

As is well known, Christian Science turns the tables on Cartesianism and argues that all disease has mental and spiritual roots. In fact, Christian Science was part of a larger development in the mid to late nineteenth century that understood physical healing as an expression of a dependence on larger spiritual forces and energies. Each person could gain access to this higher level of reality (Emerson's "oversoul," David Palmer's "Innate," Mesmerism's "animal magnetism," Phineas Quimby's "mind cure"), by removing psychological and spiritual blockages to healing. These new approaches differed in some respects from earlier health movements in that they counseled patients to gain access to an abundant and beneficent energy or spirit. This aesthetic sensibility that yearned for a kind of harmony between the person and nature contrasted with the more moralistic approaches of dietary regimes, herbalists, and advocates of hydrotherapy who argued that disease is a consequence of excessive stimulation and counseled moderation and living in accordance with God's laws. Nevertheless, both the aesthetic and ascetic branches of alternative medicine departed from the conventional medical profession in their emphasis on natural remedies, individualized treatment regimes, the self-healing capacities of the body, the democratization of expertise, and vitalism.[6]

"Regular" medicine, which, since the late eighteenth century emphasized "heroic" treatments of disease (purging, leeching, ingesting of opiates and purgatives) coexisted with the "sectarian" therapies that were less intrusive and placed a greater emphasis on "natural" remedies. Intraprofessional rivalries existed within orthodox medicine and the heterodox therapies competed in a system that was pluralistic in terms of availability in the health care market and in the sense of power and state recognition. Homeopathic medicine was a strong competitor with thirty-one journals, eighty-five local societies, seventy-four hospitals and twenty-two homeopathic colleges by 1900.[7] Various forms of botanical medicine with roots in Thomsonianism and Grahamism also flourished, appealing to segments of the working class as well as artisans and farmers who often distrusted heroic medicine (the forerunner of biomedicine). In addition, women were prominent in hydrotherapy, which emphasized the "water cure" as well as diet, rest, and exercise. Women were especially prominent in the spiritualist movement where it offered women a voice as well as a vehicle for entry into the health professions. While hydrotherapy reached the height of its popularity in the mid-nineteenth century, it experienced a revival in the 1890s when it broadened its perspective to include other natural therapies and became the forerunner of naturopathy.[8] Unlike various forms of botanical medicine, spiritualism[9] and hydrotherapy appealed predominately to the middle class.

Only in the twentieth century did biomedicine become hegemonic and gain legitimacy as coterminous with science and progress. When elite physicians transformed the previously ineffective AMA into a national professional association, reflecting their interests as well as those of major corporate-sponsored foundations and segments of the corporate capitalist class, the first step had been taken in establishing biomedical dominance. By 1901, the reorganized AMA began a process of review of medical education that culminated in the Flexner Report of 1910. This report, sponsored by the Carnegie Foundation, resulted in the denial of funding to medical schools that did not fit the bio-medical model (and were therefore deemed to be unscientific), drastically reducing the number of doctors trained by medical schools and transforming the class, ethnic, and gender character of the medical profession, making it a predominately white male, upper-middle-class profession. Moreover, the report contributed to the establishment and hegemony of the biomedical paradigm that revolved around the germ theory of disease and a reductionist model of the human body. This paradigm became the only one supported by major research foundations and granted legitimacy by the state through licensure laws. The pluralistic health care system that had existed in the nineteenth century very rapidly declined.[10]

Biomedicine understands itself as an outgrowth of scientific progress. We can interpret this claim through a version of Habermas's argument, which he appropriates from Max Weber. By differentiating the pursuit of truth from questions of justice and morality, biomedicine could develop through a learning process that did not occur in older metaphysical systems, where claims to truth and morality were not distinguished (disease could be attributed to the moral failings or spiritual pollution of the patient). When illness is attributed to moral sources, certain hypothetical questions that can be experimentally verified are excluded. If disease is a result of an occupation by a malevolent spirit, there are no conditions that would permit the falsification of such a position. As a result, there can be no learning and intellectual progress. In short, the differentiation of value spheres allows for a one-sided pursuit of truth by experts and for a learning process to develop. The gains from this pursuit of medical knowledge are made available to the public in the form of increasing life expectancy and health.[11]

Of course this understanding of biomedicine as an embodiment of the progress of science is a vast oversimplification. It excludes institutional forces that shape the nature and practice of medicine and drive it in certain directions. For example, the connection between biomedicine and prescription drugs has been shaped by the interests of pharmaceutical industries as well as science. Treatments for disease that cannot be patented and therefore cannot be a source of profit may never reach most patients or be recommended by doctors.

The relationship between medicine and the pharmaceutical industry may also be reflected in the content of medical education. Until quite recently, most medical schools taught next to nothing about nutrition or botanical medicine and its bearing upon health and well-being. Moreover, the official recognition that biomedicine achieved from the state in the form of financial subsidies and credentialization, among other things, served to exclude competitors.[12] Biomedicine, therefore, cannot be considered merely as an extension of science, simpliciter. Instead, it occupies a complex intersection between cognitive progress opened up by modern science and powerful institutional interests.

Nivarro argues that biomedicine became dominant because of its congruence with dominant sectors within corporate capitalism. Biomedicine construed disease such that the social and class dimensions were bracketed in favor of viewing disease as an individual phenomenon caused by pathogens requiring treatment by experts. In Navarro's words,

> Disease was not an outcome of specific power relations but rather a biological, individual phenomenon where the cause of disease was the immediately observable factor, the bacteria. In this redefinition, clinical medicine became the branch of scientific medicine to study the biological-individual phenomena and social medicine became that other branch of medicine, which would study the distribution of disease as the aggregate of individual phenomenon. Both branches shared the vision of disease as an alteration, a pathological change in the human body (perceived as a machine), caused by an outside agent (unicausality), or several agents (multicausality).[13]

A few examples illustrate these points. Epidemiological studies of hypertension show that there are a variety of interventions from exercise, meditation, weight loss, and diet that can have a dramatic impact on lowering blood pressure. However, as two medical doctors point out, the total research investment in nonpharmacologic approaches is, in their words,

> probably less than the cost of developing a single new drug. Meanwhile more than 200 drugs are marketed in the U.S. for the treatment of hypertension and, even government-sponsored research focuses on narrow biochemical and hormonal approaches predictably leading toward the development of further drug therapies. Within the

realm of pharmacological approaches the latitude for research is severely constrained by the imperative of corporate profitability. Thus me too drugs, minor modifications of existing best sellers represent the vast majority of the new drugs introduced. Indeed, the panoply of hypertensive drugs available present no more than 15 truly distinct agents.[14]

The same authors also point to the connection between the use of cardiac machines (automatic arrhythmia detectors), the growth of intensive care units in hospitals and the financial interests of electronic companies such as Hewlett Packert and American Optical despite the weak evidence of the overall value of these machines and units in reducing fatalities among cardiac victims.

Another example of the relationship between the corporate world and biomedicine is the close connection between the manufacturers of mammogram machines (Siemens, DuPont, General Electric, among others), the cancer drug industry, and the American Cancer Society (ACS). The companies that produce mammography equipment donate considerable funds to the ACS and have representatives on its advisory boards. Cancer drug companies such as AstraZeneca are also major financial backers of the ACS's cancer prevention programs, and AstraZeneca is also a manufacturer of industrial chemicals and pesticides. The emphasis in the ACS is on breast cancer prevention through an aggressive campaign to encourage premenopausal women to get mammograms despite the lack of evidence for its effectiveness and promoting risky "chemo prevention" drugs such as Tamoxifen. But the ACS spends less than one-one-hundredth of 1 percent of its annual budget researching environmental carcinogenesis. While more than 10 percent of adult cancer deaths are due to exposure to occupational hazards and while diet accounts for approximately one-third of all cancers, the National Cancer Institute (NCI) spends about four million dollars researching occupational exposures and educating the public about diet. This is less than 1 percent of its budget. There is certainly enough evidence to be suspicious of a cancer prevention program largely funded by chemical and pharmaceutical companies that emphasizes technologies and regimes from which it stands to profit greatly and not research and preventive measures that may threaten its interests.[15]

The emphasis upon high technology medicine (e.g., heart bypass surgery, pacemakers, and organ transplants), it has been argued, can be linked to their high cost and potential for profitability. The use of medical technology, in other words, is embedded in larger commercial and bureaucratic interests. As Levins argues,

> A hospital buys an expensive machine to attract doctors and patients. But once on hand, it has to be used. You can't allow an MRI machine to sit idle in the hospital so doctors are encouraged to use it if only amortize the institution's investment. Another is that in order to keep the "batting average" of a surgeon high, he or she has to perform enough operations (several hundred a year) to keep skill levels up. An isolated hospital with only one heart transplant every three or four months is not a safe place to go. The wise patient will seek out a hospital with a highly regarded cardiac service equipped with the latest technology. But to win that prestige, skills must be maintained, so there's an incentive to keep both surgeons and machines working.[16]

Biomedicine, in other words, is not simply an expression of scientific progress but is shaped by larger institutional factors.

According to Andre Gorz the vast majority of medical resources are used by only 4 percent of very ill patients. These patients require elaborate and complex interventions which are very costly and consistent with the overspecialization within modern medicine. Gorz argues that these interventions and their cost would be significantly reduced if more resources were devoted to prevention and more effective treatment of general health problems in the population. The processing of patients (the structure and organization of time in terms of patient care), the accessibility of medical care and its relationship to the class system, and the numbers and distribution of doctors and the kinds of specialties they practice are also market driven.[17]

The Lifeworld and Meaning

We have mentioned "lifeworld" in the context of the impoverishment of meaning. But the concept needs further clarification. The lifeworld refers to the more or less diffused and unproblematic horizons that people draw upon to come to an understanding about themselves, the world in which they live, and their modes of interaction with one another. In other words, the lifeworld is the source of cultural traditions and the basis for their renewal, as well as for integrating people into groups and transmitting competencies that are essential to the formation of a person's identity (cultural reproduction, social integration, and socialization). While aspects of the lifeworld can be called into question, for instance, by contesting assumptions about gender, the lifeworld as a whole cannot be problematized. For to do so would be to escape all intuitively certain and uncontested assumptions—which is inconceivable for the existence of any social world. Since the lifeworld is linguistically mediated, problematizing the entire lifeworld would require problematizing the entirety of the language we use. But we can only use language to explore language and therefore always remain within it.[18]

How is meaning related to the lifeworld? Meaning is connected to social interactions that renew and extend to new circumstances and problems the background assumptions in which people are embedded. We should not conflate meaning with value. Value has to do with ends or goals that can always be relativized into means for further goals in an infinite regress. Meaning, on the other hand, has to do with the actualization of potentials in the world we dwell in.[19] To illustrate the point: in some ethnic neighborhoods fishermen, after returning from a fishing trip, would distribute the catch free to their neighbors, actualizing a background of communalism and ethnic solidarity. On the other hand, if giving fish were simply a means to a subjectively constructed end, for example, to elicit indebtedness for the sake of future business plans, then fish giving would not actualize any pre-given set of assumptions (a world) and fish could be deployed in the future for other strategic purposes.

If meaning has to do with the renewal of the background, taken-for-granted assumptions in the lifeworld, then what we are really talking about here is the appropriation of the past or the relevance of the past for giving our lives significance. Meaning, in this sense, has to do with dwelling within something, in contrast to constructing or representing something for our use. The latter has to do with Heidegger's characterization of modern society as the "age of the world picture." Everything tends toward meaninglessness when it is before us and we instrumentalize it for our own purpose, but meaning increases when we actualize that which is behind us in order to address problems in the world and therefore is not completely at our disposal.[20]

There are three ways of understanding the way modern societies change our relationship to the lifeworld and lead to a loss of meaning. The first is connected to an increasingly critical stance that the modern world has toward the past. Today the past is not automatically renewed without contestation. It is critically appropriated and subject to reflection and debate. The rationalization of modern society can be understood as a process in which the lifeworld is increasingly problematized and the object of critical debate. Insofar as this rationalization process occurs, it can be argued that the past is either critically renewed or the past becomes lost and inaccessible. For example, understandings of the physical world become destabilized as they are incorporated into scientific investigation and analysis. No longer is nature an agent with goals and purposes. Instead, nature is an object of investigation, understood theoretically and controlled technologically. To the extent to which nature is part of the lifeworld and embedded in larger horizons of meaning, science disembeds it and therefore eliminates it as a resource for addressing problems in the world. In a larger sense we can see that the capacity of modern societies to engage in critical reflection on the past can serve to undermine the social certainties of religious traditions and therefore the unquestioned authority of the lifeworld. The development of modern therapy and its diffusion throughout the population problematizes questions of identity (e.g., Who am I? Where do I belong?) and as a result calls into question the possibility of coherent narratives about the self.

The second way in which modern societies change our relationship to the lifeworld is connected to the differentiation of value spheres that were once combined and undifferentiated in religious/ metaphysical systems. This differentiation leads to expert cultures that pursue one-sidedly issues in the form of truth, morality, and aesthetic expression. If we construe the rise of expert cultures as an institutional form of the critical renewal of the past, the problem becomes the mediation between these expert cultures and the lifeworld, which is increasingly detached from the progress taking place in these spheres. In Habermas's terms, the growth of science, modern law, and the progress of art must be reintegrated into the experiences of everyday actors. If this is not done, the lifeworld suffers from anomie or a loss of direction.

Finally, there is what Habermas calls the colonization of the lifeworld or how institutional imperatives organized through the media of money and power reify social interactions and evacuate them of meaning. Here people's interactions become coordinated in ways that are beyond their understanding and participation. In Habermas's terms coordination is "delinguistified" or separated from the communicative efforts of participants.[21]

This process of undermining the certainties of the past leads to a series of paradoxes. The growing critical appropriation of the past becomes an opportunity to remove prejudices, dogmatism, and unjust power relations that are part of traditional practices, that is, the lifeworld. The rise of expert cultures permits advances in the cognitive, moral, and expressive spheres of life. The rise of institutional structures such as the modern state and economy provides relief from the need to reach agreement for the coordination of social interactions. Yet, these processes threaten to undermine the substance of tradition and therefore dissolve meaning so that we arrive at what Walter Benjamin feared would be a meaningless emancipation.[22] In this book, as we examine modern medicine and its alternatives, we want to stay within the framework of these paradoxes, which Habermas argues is the source of the most fruitful encounter with the present.

How is modern medicine situated in relationship to these threats to meaning and the disintegration of the continuities of the past? We take this question seriously because we want to argue along with Benjamin that meaning and happiness are bound to the renewal of tradition or what he called the process of secular illumination. Habermas puts it this way: "We need those rescued semantic potentials if we are to interpret the world in terms of our own needs and only if the source of these potentials does not run dry can the claim to happiness be fulfilled."[23]

Medicine and the Lifeworld

Modern medicine contributes to the depletion of meaning in the lifeworld because of the problem of mediating its language and practices with that of patients. We explore this through an examination of the medical view of the person as a biological system and medical practices that incorporate this understanding. In biomedicine the body is sectioned off into distinct subsystems and layers and described in technical language to allow for interventions. These interventions become the source for research leading to new diagnostic procedures, drugs, and surgical techniques. There is, in addition, a commitment in medicine to life in itself as a value, independent of its significance for the person. This leads to the commitment to prolonging life through extraordinary means. The maintenance of the biological system is the highest value. This decoupling of the body from the lifeworld is instantiated in a range of daily medical practices which medical science attempts to validate. One neurooncologist we interviewed captures the medical abstraction of the body from the lifeworld in a particularly graphic reflection on the worth and relevance of alternative medicine:

I think that there is . . . um . . . a valid aspect [to alternative medicine] in the sense that . . . the valid aspect to it, I think, comes out of holistic medicine is to treat a person rather than a disease. Um . . . and to which I say that's . . . that's very important when you're not successful in treating the disease. The patients don't want holistic care. They want to be better, okay? They don't . . . they don't need a partner in their life, you know, managing it. They want someone to cure the problem. I can give, again, an example . . . you take your car to a dealership and the transmission's not shifting into high gear and he says, "Well, I can't do anything about it but I'm gonna help you deal with that emotionally." You'll say, "No thanks, I want someone to put my transmission into high gear." It's the same with . . . I always say you don't need any psycho-social management, you don't need any art of medicine, you don't need holistic . . . if you were a hundred percent successful.

To become a doctor, a student must learn how to characterize patients through what Good calls the "write-up" and to communicate the content of that write-up to senior staff through a convincing diagnosis.[24] They must also learn a kind of abridged form of communication with patients that is enforced through medical authority. This abridgment is necessitated by the structure of medical time; the daily rounds that leave no time for open and textured dialogue. In a medical write-up, the patient's medical problem and history is presented concisely and in technical language. The patient's life history, religious beliefs, emotional state, cultural background, and social relationships are bracketed. If any of this is included in presentations to senior staff, interns find out quickly that they are violating medical/diagnostic norms. The more interesting and complex the case, and the longer it takes to make a definitive diagnosis, the greater the approval of colleagues. As one doctor put it,

My intern always used to say . . . a good case is where you don't make the diagnosis for an hour. A great case is where you don't make the diagnosis for a day. But if it takes a week to make a diagnosis, now that's what we call a fascinoma.[25]

One physician who later became interested in Native American healing practices described the fascination with diagnosis in his medical training in the following way.

The great thrill for most of my teachers was in diagnosis. As one neurology professor said, "Most patients are very boring. What is interesting is what they might have and making sure they don't have it. What is left after that—the treatment and so on—is either boring or difficult. Few diseases respond in the textbook manner to the drugs we offer them. Some diseases respond to no drugs. Invariably, patients never do exactly as they are told. Patients have the pesky habit of doing what they want, regardless of our advice."[26]

When we combine these stories with the research demonstrating that doctors spend little time communicating with patients, it is clear that the time spent in diagnosing patients is a component of a self-referential, technical language that is divorced from the everyday language of patients.[27]

The emphasis on diagnosis intensifies the distance that separates the doctor from the patient. This is reinforced by studies of the content of doctor-patient communication. For instance, one study of patients in England concludes that the rules of communication between doctors and patients differ from rules of everyday communication. Doctor-patient communication is based on what this study calls a perspective difference. Doctors see patients as typical cases and apply rules and categories that they learn in medical training, which occlude the subjective experience of discomfort, pain, and fear. Moreover, the normal interactional rules of everyday communication are broken because communication between doctors and patients is one-way and decontextualized. Finally, patients' accounts of their illnesses are devalued and even omitted.[28]

This process is sometimes actively pursued by patients who seek to be relieved of responsibility for the understanding and treatment of their own illness by seeing themselves from the point of view of the "voice of the doctor." [29] In one study of the language ("chart talk") used by occupational therapists and nurses in formal settings, this perspective difference between patients and the medical world is captured:

Sandra (OT): Is OT needed?
Nurse: Ah, no, just PT, well . . .
Sandra: What's the diagnosis?
Nurse: Left CVA [cerebral vascular accident] with right residual.
Sandra: Any problems with his speech?
Nurse: No, none.
Sandra: What's his right upper extension like?
Nurse: He's functional, but can't really use his fingers.
Sandra: Can you also request an OT consult? He needs one.

Nurse: OK.
Sandra: Does he have the ability to do ADLs [Activities of Daily Living]?
Nurse: Yes. We try to put washcloths in his hands.
Sandra: You might try AB pads.[30]

Even when doctors would like to reduce the marginality of patients it is difficult for them to do so because, as one writer notes,

> [T]hey [doctors] have been trained to diagnose and discuss syndromes in a precise terminology in which they can readily communicate with their peers. This discourse unites medical professionals and at the same time alienates the uninitiated so that access to this language becomes a tool of empowerment. Perri Klass recalls how she picked up "endless jargon," as well as "the patterns of speech and grammatical conventions," during the first three months she worked in a hospital as a medical student. "This special language," she comments, "contributes to a sense of closeness and professional spirit among people who are under a great deal of stress." The converse to that closeness is the exclusion of those unable to understand this parlance, so that in effect a barrier is erected between lay people and those who have undergone medical training.[31]

In light of all of this, what do we make of Habermas's argument that the depletion of meaning in the lifeworld can only be arrested through the translation of the gains of expert knowledge into the communicative practices of everyday life? While this project of mediation may be more plausible in other expert domains, such as the translation of art criticism to a wider public in developing aesthetic appreciation or in morality through the medium of law and moral education, it's hard to see how the biomedical language of allopathic medicine can be translated into everyday life and form the basis for a narrative reconstruction of personal life. When such translations occur, they usually push people to the margins of medical institutions. This is Mattingly's conclusion in her study of the talk of occupational therapists, who in formal settings display "chart talk" while narrative story telling about patients takes place in elevators, cafeterias, and at parties.

Part of the difficulty of translation has to do with institutional interests and the way technical language legitimates the power of doctors over patients. In other technical areas such as architecture, law, and academic research and teaching (and, as we will argue later, in alternative health), professional work must be translated back and forth from lifeworld to expert culture if it is to go on at all. Architects cannot reconstruct the physical environment of people without some translation into their value system and purposes, whether those are manipulated or not. College professors engage in some translation through participating in teaching and research that is accessible to the public. Modern law is grounded in the consent and participation of the larger community and ultimately must rest on their values. But the very nature of medicine, the treatment of illness, requires distance from the patient's lifeworld in terms of both the language of medicine and the interests of doctors. The object of medicine is not the person but the body construed as a physical system operating independent of the will and purposes of the subject, yet the paradox of illness is that it reaches into the totality of a person's life. But the medical model cannot acknowledge this and remain what it is.

The depletion of meaning that is a byproduct of the rise of expert cultures is internally connected to the colonization of the lifeworld. Colonization, as discussed earlier, refers to the coordination of action independent of the communicative efforts of participants in the lifeworld. Coordination, in this sense, is delinguistified; it happens behind people's backs. This is a process that can be analytically distinguished from the rise of expert cultures based on the rationalization of the lifeworld. At least according to Habermas, the rise of expert cultures raises the question of cultural transmission between experts and everyday actors that can theoretically happen in a balanced and fruitful way. On the other hand, colonization refers to the intrusion of system imperatives in a domain that produces pathologies, that is, the lifeworld, which should only be reproduced by the communicative efforts of actors. The system cannot replace the efforts of people to understand themselves, to morally relate to one another, and to express their own desires and needs. Otherwise, there will result an increase in social pathologies ranging from anomie to subjective emptiness. The driving force in colonization is institutional interests and their own reproduction rather than the sharing of intellectual, moral, and aesthetic gains that derive from expert cultures.[32]

We can clarify the modalities of medical colonization through the use of Lukes's classification of the different modes of the deployment of power.[33] First, there is the direct exercise of power by one actor over another through an overt decision. For example, the doctor may decide on a medical strategy of dealing with an illness and the patient, despite misgivings, follows the protocol. Since doctors cannot in practice order patients to follow a protocol this form of power is rarely deployed in the medical sphere. Second, the doctor achieves compliance by not informing patients of alternatives to the recommended protocol, and the patient's decision is based on limited alternatives through medical agenda setting. The third form of power is the most subtle and reaches deepest into the texture of everyday life. Here, patients deceive themselves about the efficacy of the recommended protocol because of the legitimacy of the medical profession or because of the relief of responsibility for her own treatment that the medical model provides. The latter two expressions of power are examples of distorted communication because doctors' institutional interest in reproducing the medical system is hidden in a technical, objectivistic language.

The process of colonization is revealed in an examination of doctor-patient interactions. Those interactions reveal the operation of power in terms of self-deception on the part of both patient and doctor. Both forms of self-deception are the conditions for the impersonal coordination of action by the medical system. As Anspach and others have shown, a central feature of medical education is the case presentation.[34] Here interns and residents learn to interpret their own activity not as an investigative art form but as an impersonal outcome of diagnostic technology. For example, "Auscultation of the head revealed a very large bruit, and angiography showed a very large arteriovenous malformation in the head. . . ."[35] Here the deception is that doctors do not need to interpret the data. Instead, the machines themselves reveal the accurate diagnosis of which the doctor is a passive transmitter. Just as the doctor transmits the authoritative judgments of medical technology, so too when interns and residents communicate through case presentations and write-ups, their own agency is suppressed. So, for example, "No betamethasome was given" is the standard rather than "Dr. _____ gave no betamethasome."[36]

The impersonal coordination of doctors by the medical system becomes the basis for the extension of the system into the lifeworld. What doctors do to themselves, they then do to patients. The central purpose of doctor-patient communication is to convince the patient to see herself in terms of the language of the write-up (or case presentation), as a biological system in need of repair from medical expertise. This is how we can understand the notion of "medical compliance." The person becomes voluntarily absorbed into the medical system and detached from the lifeworld. When patients see themselves as medical objects, we have an instance of "reification," the relational character of human life is severed and transformed into a "thinglike" state. Illness becomes subjectively meaningless, an occupation by enemy forces that can refer not only to the disease but also in some cases the medical system itself.

One doctor we interviewed, a leading critic of alternative medicine, described the experiences of his father, who had open-heart surgery:

> My father had open-heart surgery. He saw his surgeon one time after his surgery. I said, "Did that bother you [that the doctor did not develop a relationship with the father]?" I mean that's typical for cardiacs, you know, I mean the residents saw him and stuff, he said, "Hi," to my dad, "Hi, Frank, how you doing?" Okay. He never saw him again. I asked him [Frank], "Does that bother you?" He said, "I don't give a crap. He made me feel better. My chest doesn't hurt any more and I can go out and play golf and do all this stuff and I feel great. So, I don't care who he is or . . . I don't care if I couldn't recognize him." That's the point. The same way with our tumor patients. If they came in here with malignant tumors and I could say, "Here take this pill, and you're now [cured],". . . I could insult them, I could call their wives whores, I could do anything that you wanted, they wouldn't care because I took the cancer away.

Here is a good example of a patient seeing himself in terms of the language of the medical system and its reifying character. In this sense, the self-understanding of "cure" does not involve a transformation of the self in relation to the lifeworld but an external intervention that happens mechanically. A person is cured the way a car with transmission problems is repaired.

Another illustration can be found in the extensive literature on the experiences of women in childbirth. In the work of Graham and Oakley obstetricians and mothers often have conflicting frames of reference on reproduction.[37] Doctors view childbirth as potentially pathological, while women see this as "natural." Doctors view themselves as having a monopoly on knowledge about childbirth while women see themselves as having valuable knowledge as women. The last two factors relate to questions of control and communication;

> [W]omen typically wish to retain control over what happens, especially during childbirth. Physicians usually act as if all the key decisions are for them to take. Some women resent the use of technology during childbirth because it involves a loss of personal control and

clashes with their perception of childbirth as an essentially normal process. Physicians see technology as an important resource in containing a potentially pathological process. And fourth, women often complain about unsatisfactory communication. Questions are difficult to ask and, if asked, are frequently ignored or interpreted as requests for reassurance. Physicians tend to perceive mothers' questions as evidence of anxiety rather than requests for information, and either fail to respond at all or resort to vague or trivial answers if pressed.[38]

Of course, much has changed since this research was conducted, but this does not change our principal argument. The lifeworld of the person is detached step by step from the person so that the person can become a medical patient. It's an empirical question as to the degree to which a particular person resists or succumbs to this process.

The fundamental expression of this absorption of the patient's lifeworld into the "medical body" occurs among terminally ill patients who seek medical intervention. It is fundamental because it is here where the person is most thoroughly captured by the medical system. Cancer patients often receive "chemotherapy" between other treatments and with the proliferation of various forms of cancer, experience with chemotherapy is quite common. What is the lived experience of this treatment? According to Arthur Frank, chemotherapy patients experience a peculiar psychological state he calls "embodied paranoia." Patients begin to fear the very agents who ostensibly exist to make them well. In fact, these agents are instruments of perceived torture. They transform the body from an instrument of involvement in the world to an object of continuous pain that blocks connections to oneself and other people.[39] This is analogous to what Scarry calls the "process of deworlding" among torture victims.[40] But, unlike torture victims, chemotherapy patients do not have clear objects toward which to direct their anger and hatred. Instead they drift in a state of bewilderment and confusion. In most cases, patients believe their doctors are well intentioned but feel themselves to be victims of a system and its required protocols.

Alternative Health and the Mediation of Expertise

Alternative health cannot be equated in a simple sense with folk medicine since it is bound up with modern society and the rise of expert cultures (not to mention the commodification of their services).

Alternative health has its schools in which practitioners are trained, where there is clearly a body of knowledge that is transmitted, the mastery of which is recognized through the granting of degrees. Credentialized experts in various alternative health fields provide services for fees, petition for state recognition, desire reimbursement from insurance companies, and call themselves health professionals.[41] Yet, alternative health has a strikingly different relationship to the lifeworld than that of biomedicine.

Biomedicine originates in institutional research funded by the state, universities, and the corporate sector. While biomedicine scours traditional societies for new drugs, the pathways to the natural world are erased through the industrial processing of the product and genetic manipulation of the natural substance. In contrast, the knowledge transmitted in alternative health schools is a reworking of health traditions that originate in some cases in the premodern world. The knowledge and the products that are studied and utilized in alternative health do not originate in scientific laboratories or pharmaceutical companies but instead are embedded in forms of life. For example, many forms of acupuncture practiced in this country derive from Chinese traditional medicine and the world view that informs it. Myotherapy, a bodywork specialty widely employed by alternative massage therapists, is based on a traditional Japanese form of massage—Shiatsu. Herbal treatments are embedded in traditional medical systems such as Ayurvedic, Native American healing practices, nineteenth-century American botanical medicine, and traditional Chinese medicine.

One practitioner, who practices energy field work in conjunction with various forms of massage, explained that the roots of his expertise derive from traditional Christian healing practices, "the laying on of hands," which "was an integral part of the early Church."

> This was something that if you were a minister in the year sixty AD, this was part of what you did, but now it's . . . If you go into the average Methodist or Presbyterian church and talk about the fact that you do this, it's like this wall goes up. If they're Presbyterian or Methodist, they just decide that you're nuts that you need to be restrained.

Practitioners of "alternative forms of massage" and energy manipulation may understand their practices as a recovery and extension of religious healing traditions that were embedded in the lifeworld of traditional communities.

Even when these treatments are lifted, partially transformed, and eclectically combined in alternative health schools, the point remains that they originate in the lifeworld and retain deep connections to it. Unlike biomedicine in which pharmaceuticals are industrially processed, genetically rearranged, and patented in the form of intellectual property, alternative health treatments are not filtered in this way nor can they be patented since herbs, organic food, and "energy fields" remain common resources of humanity. Even though alternative health products and practices are mediated in a variety of ways through schooling and the acquisition of expertise, they can still be reabsorbed and grounded in ongoing social practices.

A few examples will illustrate our point. One elderly women we interviewed was a founder of the Natural Living Group (NLG), organized to share nutritional information and organic food in the context of ongoing community events, weekly meetings (where lectures disseminate information about alternative nutrition and healing techniques), and organic food festivals. Living in a rural area, the founders of this group pooled information from their own gardening activities, knowledge of organic farming (one member grew up on a dairy farm) and nutrition, to address the health problems of people in the community. In the words of one member, "We shared produce and shared ideas." For the NLG, health was connected to the lifeworld in two ways: one was through the transmission of practices from their own past and the other through the mediation of knowledge filtered through expert systems. The transmission in both directions, vertically (from alternative health experts) and horizontally (from generation to generation) tends to be reinforcing and complementary.

Weekly lectures in the local Pittsburgh food co-op, macrobiotic study groups, vegetarian cooking classes, alternative cancer groups, are all examples of the incorporation of semidetached expert systems into the practices of groups in the lifeworld. Macrobiotics, a traditional Japanese-derived nutritional regime, is studied monthly in various homes based on assigned readings over herbal tea and organic desert. The discussion begins with the reading and then ranges over broader social and political questions. The Committee for Freedom of Choice in Cancer Therapy (CFC) provides monthly lectures on unconventional treatments for cancer and other chronic diseases. At these events, community groups, national alternative health organizations (such as the National Health Federation), and local health stores provide organic food, reading material, informational videos, health information and anecdotal information about the experiences of patients with chronic diseases. Here we can see the embeddedness of alternative health even when it is filtered through some form of expertise.

Expertise in alternative health is compromised because this expertise can be more easily absorbed into the competencies of actors in everyday life. People are not just subjected to alternative health. They master the information and protocols and expand their own individual skills. This is why the gap between expert and patient is more fluid and indeterminate in alternative health than in biomedicine. The skills in food combining, juicing, use of herbal teas, bach flower essences, oxygen protocols acquired by patients become part of the texture of their lives. As we will argue later, alternative health becomes part of a technology of the self.

Alternative practitioners tend to encourage their own marginalization. Many of the speakers at the CFC are not credentialized but seem to have mastered a body of knowledge and practice that they offer others to incorporate in their lives. An Amish healer, who runs a health food store in Ohio, gave a CFC lecture on oxidation treatments for intestinal disorders ranging from ulcers to parasites. His knowledge came from his practices as a healer in the Amish community but also his experiences in alternative health conferences and in his capacity as health store owner. We find here that credentialized health practitioners and others who claim expertise mix freely in various programs without tension and without a sense of threat to the health practitioners. Patients, who seek alternative treatments for chronic diseases, often become advocates of alternative medicine and appear in various settings as experts and in some cases write books about their experiences. As a result, in alternative health the boundary between health professionals and patients is not as clear as it is in biomedicine.

One prominent personality in the alternative health movement, Maureen Solomon, manages and finances her own alternative health research organization. Her organization researches scientific journals, publicizes the experiences and innovations of alternative health practitioners, making it available in the form of newsletters, nationwide lecture appearances, and in popular books. She appears regularly on a Christian TV station, answering phone-in questions, using anecdotal examples as well as research from her own organization. Solomon is an expert but without formal credentials.

The AIDS epidemic and responses to it by the gay community graphically illustrates the difference in transmissability of expertise in alternative compared to biomedicine. As O'Connor demonstrates, PWAs (people with AIDS) have created alternative health networks that disseminate a wide range of information about alternative treatments for AIDS.[42] There exist in gay communities dense networks of partnership, aid and communication that incorporate the entire range of alternative protocols from metaphysical approaches like Reiki to Chinese herbal treatments and acupuncture to megavitamin approaches. Moreover, people learn and transform these protocols through their own practices. One cannot conceive of how such a process of transmission could take place with respect to biomedicine. AIDS patients would have to go to medical school in order to be able to treat themselves, but in the process they would detach themselves from the ongoing interactions of the community and its associations with wider lifeworld practices.

As we have discussed, the compromised nature of expertise in alternative health and the way it makes more porous the boundaries between professionals and laypeople suggests an example of a successful mediation between specialized circles of knowledge and the practice of actors in the lifeworld. Habermas raised the problem of mediation in modern societies but he could find few examples of where expertise and everyday actors mutually transform one another. Alternative health offers perhaps the clearest model of what successful mediation of expertise might look like and therefore provides the grounds for believing it is possible in other areas.

Meaning or Cure?

Weber argued that the price of progress is the disenchantment of the world. In other words, the process of societal rationalization has resulted in the collapse of religious and metaphysical systems that provided coherent answers to the contingencies of life. Birth, illness, accidents, and death become arbitrary and meaningless experiences, no longer understood in terms of our place in the world. They confront us as arbitrary facts that we have to face but cannot be accounted for in terms of any ultimate significance. While religious and metaphysical systems may continue in the life experiences of specific groups, they no longer serve as an orientation for society as a whole, a public source of meaning. The condition of the modern world produces a separation between truth and consolation—what is in fact happening in the world around us and what our heart wishes to be the case. The pursuit of truth becomes the domain of science that does not tell us how to live.

Biomedicine can be situated in the context of this dilemma. Perhaps the price we pay for its increasing efficacy is the loss of coherent narratives about the self in relation to illness. In this sense, the best we can do, in the spirit of Weber, is to confront heroically the breakdown of the body from the point of view of its ultimate meaninglessness. Illness provides for all of us a personal experience with disenchantment as it operates in everyday life. As Giddens maintains, the process of disenchantment transforms the character of everyday life. Everyday life now is governed by routines or an architecture of habits. Routines are social practices no longer referred to or justified by fundamental moral horizons.[43] Therefore, when tragedy or crisis strikes, routines fall apart leaving the person disoriented and without support. The ill person can no longer call upon the practices of everyday life to comprehend why she is ill. If illness is merely the breakdown of the body disembedded from morally grounded social practices, the round of daily habits cannot hide the disenchantment of life. In this sense modern medicine contributes at the most intimate level to a deepening of the experience of disenchantment.

The meaninglessness of illness may be compounded by the fact that biomedicine's interventions are less effective in the context of a range of chronic diseases—allergies, cancer, Chronic Fatigue Syndrome, Crohn's, MS, lupus, among others. As a result, the loss of meaning may not be even compensated by the effectiveness of medical interventions. To rephrase the neurooncologist quoted earlier, not only does medicine not offer emotional consolation for your "transmission not working" but also experts find it more and more difficult to fix it. In fact, with iatrogenesis (doctor induced illness), modern medicine may even be the source of the transmission problems. Of course, all of this can be disputed, but the fact that these questions are even being posed in light of the increasing popularity of alternative medicine, shows that these claims cannot easily be dismissed as irrational and without substance.

Alternative health can be conceptualized as an attempt to reintegrate meaning and effectiveness with respect to health and illness in the modern world. Alternative health is part of an effort to reenchant the world, an effort that involves reembedding illness in the totality of life. Enchantment has many forms and is sweeping over the entire culture. Elements of the ecology movement, feminist and men's movements (mythopoetic), the rise of the occult and New Age spirituality, popular interest in angels, near death experiences, astrology are all examples.[44] Alternative health is part of this larger phenomenon but participates in it in a unique way. Not only does alternative health seek to reembed illness in the lifeworld but it makes claims to successfully cure or heal chronic diseases in a way that competes with the hegemonic status of biomedicine. Therefore, it seeks to reunite enchantment without the loss of technical effectiveness and as a result is unwilling to make the separation that Weber said was inevitable.

Yet, this claim to reintegrate enchantment and effectiveness is not without its own limitations. Reenchantment is always partial and unstable while claims of effectiveness can be contested and in some cases may be fraudulent. These questions, of the relation between meaning and practical efficacy, that are central to the modern world, are perhaps best raised through an examination of the crisis of health and illness. Illness, after all, disrupts the ongoing continuity of social life and therefore raises poignantly fundamental questions about who we are and what our place is in the world.

CHAPTER 3

Between the Aura
and the Commodity

In the previous chapter we argued that alternative health could be understood as a response to disenchantment and the way biomedicine participates in it. Disenchantment refers to the separation of everyday life from larger horizons of meaning that serve to orient people. Biomedicine, as we have seen, intensifies this process by separating the patient from the lifeworld through its construction of the body as a physical system subject to expert intervention. We will examine in this chapter the alternative health networks we've studied in order to illuminate the ways in which alternative health communities attempt to reembed the patient in the lifeworld and in this sense reenchant social life.

As we have noted, meaning is constituted by the recovery and transmission of the semantic potentials that are embedded in the past. To reenchant reality, then, would be to draw upon traditions in ways that are relevant to the present in order to address problems as they emerge in the lifeworld. The answer, in a world where it is increasingly difficult to appropriate traditions holistically, cannot be the recovery of traditions that answer all of life's questions. How, then, is the past a resource for reenchantment with respect to life's contingencies, especially illness and suffering?

Art Sutton, as well as most of the other people we interviewed, entered alternative health because of a life crisis or illness interrupting the progress of lives that had, in many cases, been quite conventional prior to this experience. For Art, founder of Holistic Living Quest, it was his divorce that led him to travel throughout the world, looking for answers in various religious and spiritual traditions. When he returned, it was a mystical experience at a New Thought theology school that opened up for him a new direction in his life. Emily, a friend of Ed Watkowsky, has been an activist in the Natural Living Group for many decades and describes herself as a "conservative Christian." She became active in alternative health as a result of problems she experienced during the pregnancy of her first child. This led to an association with a local chiropractor and his health-oriented study group, which, in turn, sparked an interest in the environmental movement and various Eastern therapies such as meditation and acupuncture. She believes that as a nation we need to change the way we grow food, returning to methods of agriculture that were common in the farming community where she grew up. Emily is a member of the Western Pennsylvania Solar Energy Society and teaches courses at a community college on how to live more simply. She is also a devout Christian who believes that the world will soon witness the second coming of Christ and combines eclectically these religious beliefs with interests in Eastern therapies and organic farming. For Emily as well as Art, fragments of the past provided resources that helped them to give their lives a new sense of meaning. For Art, these tradition fragments came largely from eastern religion and other mystical traditions while for Emily they came largely from the farming community where she grew up.

For others whose stories we will learn about in this chapter, conventional careers and lives were reevaluated in moments of crisis, experiences that led to a critical reexamination of their past, and more often than not, aspects of modern societies. We discovered that what sustains involvement in alternative health networks are the rich, though fragmentary associations with spiritual, healing and other traditions. These connections with the past, to be discussed throughout this chapter, embed lives in a larger horizon of meaning and infuse alternative health with a weak sense of utopia. Preparing and drinking herbal tea, shopping at the food-coop, taking a meditation class, preparing macrobiotic meals, all involve a ritualized encounter with fragments of other traditions, providing a weak source of meaning and enchanting elements of everyday life. It is this experientially based appropriation of the past, neglected by many who write about alternative health, that can go a long way in explaining its attraction to such a large sector of the educated middle class.

We find the writings of Walter Benjamin of special relevance in explaining the use of the past as a source of meaning and utopian energy in alternative health. Benjamin asked, among other things, what are the sources of resistance and happiness in a world of empty progress and homogenization of experience?[1] Benjamin conceived of happiness as the experience of interruption through which the semantic potentials embedded in prior worlds are renewed. For Benjamin,[2] the modern world severs the person from the totality of life. In other words, individual biography and the course of the world move along separate paths. Weber also argues that in the modern world the experiences of people become discontinuous and no longer provide sources of wisdom that link generations.[3] At one time social life could be characterized as a circle; generations were linked through a common path of experiences and as a result wisdom could be transmitted from the older to the younger. Societal rationalization destroys the circle and fragments experience. Benjamin accepts this analysis but responds to it in a unique way. Since meaning is no longer lived and continuous with the flow of life, it has to be redeemed through flashes of memory, which interrupt the present. Memory is a process of reexperiencing the circle of life in momentary flashes.

Unlike Marx, Benjamin did not want to ride the tide of history; he wanted to resist it ("brush history against the grain").[4] In other words, happiness is not a consequence of riding the train of history into the future but more like reaching for the emergency brake. The flow of time in the present is stopped through flashes of memory that break through, like the messiah, into the endless duplication of empty strings of experience, the quantitative expansion of wealth without a corresponding qualitative deepening of happiness and well-being.[5] Capitalist modernization not only homogenizes experience, but makes the past available only in the form of ruins or fragments of practices, experiences and objects that are broken from the larger totality. These ruins by their very meaninglessness call forth the work of the allegorist to redeem and reanimate them through the work of interpretation.[6] The focus on what is empty of significance provokes the impulse for redemption.[7]

The Aura and Alternative Health

The breaking through of the past into the present is also central to Benjamin's concept of the aura.[8] The aura is the vapors or associations that surround objects and give them unique identities. The aura suggests specific worlds that the person notices through the ritualized encounter with the object. Benjamin wrote about the aura in connection with the encounter with art objects when they were embedded in religious rituals and practices and in a more subdued form when art objects are displayed in museums as unique and irreplaceable. For Benjamin the experience of the aura is an experience of looking at an object and having it look back at you. What comes through the object are the rich associations and embedded horizons of specific worlds. In this sense the aura expands the model of intersubjectivity beyond social relations to the larger world of objects and nature.

Once objects and experiences in the world are understood as partners in communication, the horizon of sympathy between the self and the world radically expands. The aura, in other words, is a way of experiencing what to Benjamin is the most fundamental drive in human existence—the drive to become identical to the world. This, for Benjamin, is the source of the energies that are released into art, language, and the messianic promise. Through the word and the image we seek correspondences with the world. The aura allows us to experience these correspondences in flashes of illumination.[9] It is this experientially based encounter that provides the energy out of which we can fashion new selves and meaningful relationships to the world. To Benjamin the point was to release the semantic energies established in this correspondence between the natural world and human beings into the larger culture for purposes of transformation. This is the achievement of interpretation. In other words, an epiphany that creates meaning has to be retrieved through interpretation and made available for the transformation of social practice.

In the world of alternative health, herbs, organic food, meditation, styles of dress, physical structures such as food co-ops and health fairs suggest associations that contrast with the commodity form. Objects such as herbs, organic food, bach flower remedies, mineral bath oils, have the auratic suggestion of traditional worlds, from indigenous cultures in the Americas and elsewhere to Eastern religions. To use an herb is not simply to ingest a product with medical properties but at the same time to partake, even if tenuously, of other times and other practices. On the label of a bottle of an herbal dietary supplement called "Cat's Claw," the following description can be found;

> Cat's Claw . . . a woody vine that grows wild in the Peruvian rain
> forest will often grow to be more than 100 feet in length. Indigenous

people of South America use this herb for a number of health related problems. Cat's Claw is another pertinent example of the new herbs being discovered in rain forest jungles. Be active in the fight to protect these rich and important regions of plant life.

Another label, for Organic Bancha Green Tea, reads,

> Eden Organic Bancha Tea is a refreshing, authentic, traditional tea. It is grown, tended, harvested and prepared exactly as it has been for centuries. Commercial teas are dyed and are poor reflections of the TEAS that became integral to cultures around the world. Bancha Tea will reward you with the essence of tea's natural character and perpetual popularity.

These auratic associations are carried over into everyday life in the form of memories and personal attachments. Here one herbal tea enthusiast describes what preparing tea means to her:

> I enjoy using the fresh herbs. When I make it myself, I know the herbs are fresh. And I enjoy using it myself and I enjoy reading about the herbs and their various uses. It kind of brings me back to an earlier, simpler time when people used herbs medicinally as well as Native Americans using them for many purposes . . . I like making herbal teas for my friends. They might have different complaints and ailments. I like being able to help them with something that's natural and is not going to harm them . . .

The auratic experience finds its most concentrated expression in the concept of the "natural." Nature and tradition are closely associated reference points in alternative health that continuously refer to one another. Traditional worlds are thought to be closer to and more in harmony with nature and its rhythms. In fact, it could be argued that nature serves as a functional equivalent for tradition among alternative health patients and practitioners. Nature invokes friendly forms of life that are on the side of the health and well-being of the person.

On another level, the identification with the natural is consistent with the quotation of traditional societies in the social practices of alternative health. Traditional societies are thought to be closer to nature and less manufactured. In this context "the natural" and traditional societies connote safety and security, simplicity, the slowing down of time, and a sense of a world threatened by the forces of progress. In other words, assorted traditions are selectively appropriated as a vehicle for attaining a more natural condition.

The natural on the most obvious level is that which is unprocessed and at one with the rhythm of life. One newsletter for the NLG contained the following description:

> We are organized to learn, share information and develop sources of help for simple, natural lifestyles. We were first organized in 1958 as the . . . Natural Foods Group. In 1986 the name was changed to . . . Natural Living Group to reflect our expanded interest into the areas of exercise, health care and the environment. We believe in a balanced diet with as many whole foods as possible, in their natural state, grown organically, and without poisonous sprays. We try to avoid refined grain products, highly processed foods and meats with hormones and antibiotics. We are concerned with whole soil, whole food, and whole people.

Organic vegetables are "natural" in that the soil used is not subject to industrial inputs—pesticides and herbicides. Herbs, which grow wild and which are the medicine provided by nature, are "natural" in contrast to pharmaceutical drugs. Deep breathing as a route to relaxation is natural in that it establishes a correspondence between the person and her environment. Deep breathing, eating organic food, and ingesting herbs are instances of a process of reconciliation between the self and the world. Rather than dominating the world, the point is to duplicate its rhythms, textures, and offerings.

Here we can see that the drive, as Benjamin pointed out, is to become identical with the world itself ("the mimetic faculty").[10] The drive to instantiate nature through bodily practices is an illustration of what Benjamin calls sensuous correspondences between the self and the world. The mimetic faculty, Benjamin claims, is even at the root of the origin of language, which continues the drive for a correspondence with the natural world but now at a nonsensuous level.[11] The language of alternative health continues this drive for correspondence through the quotation of the past.

The enemy of nature is understood to be the one-sided development of modern life, what others have called instrumental rationality, a completely manufactured and administered world. Progress, as understood by alternative health practitioners and activists, is a danger to health and to the possibility of a meaningful life. The fear of new deadly microorganisms that mutate in response to medical intervention (antibiotics) and the fear of serious ecological and health consequences of industrial farming suggests a language of catastrophe that runs through alternative health. For example, advocates of oxidation therapy assert that oxygen depletion caused by industrial pollution is now reaching dangerous levels that threaten the very survival of the species. Warren J. Belasco in his history of the alternative food movement documents how the organizers of food co-ops in the 1970s were reacting to the sense that processed foods and environmental pollutants were poisoning America. Unless Americans ate differently and treated the natural world with more care, the species was doomed. An article in the *Whole Earth Catalog* put it this way:

> It has occurred to me that if I were a dictator determined to control the national press, *Organic Gardening* would be the first publication I'd squash, because it's the most subversive. I believe that organic gardeners are in the forefront of a serious effort to save the world by changing man's orientation to it, to move away from the collective, centrist, superindustrial state, toward a simpler, realer one-to-one relationship with the earth itself.[12]

Paul Ehrlich, in *The Population Bomb,* presented a radical form of this sentiment that was pervasive during that period and can still find echoes today:

> We must realize that unless we are extremely lucky, everybody will disappear in a cloud of blue steam in twenty years. . . . Some people are beginning to suspect that due to a lack of interest, tomorrow has been canceled.[13]

This does not mean that alternative health practitioners are pessimistic. Instead, they have a limited confidence in the capacity of their own protocols and the consciousness that suffuses them to counteract these macrohistorical trends. The transformation of individual consciousness and practices is sometimes seen as a source and expression of a world-transforming global change. Unlike the early period of the alternative food movement, the later New Age avatars are found of predicting a new global consciousness (a "harmonic convergence") where the totality of life will be transfigured.[14]

On a more cultural level, progress suggests the proliferation of the commodity form and its devaluation of the lifeworld. Many of the practitioners and activists we interviewed complained that people are so busy making a living and spending money that the point of their lives is no longer clear. One practitioner observed that there are positive changes in American culture in the form of resistance to the anesthetizing impact of modern life and its commitment to progress. Nevertheless, he observes that many people remain anesthetized.

> I think there are some forces that work against [positive change]. There are elements of the population that get more and more meshed in what I call anesthesia activities, television, computer games, that sort of thing. So, there's certainly an element of the population that is not participating in any kind of shift. They are very much wrapped up in their bread and circuses. They make their living, come home and turn on the T.V., and then they don't have to think any more . . .

Eileen, a co-op staff member opposes any effort to modernize the co-op by increasing product choice and making deliveries of goods and services more efficient, as if the co-op was in competition with supermarkets.

> I'm against progress. I think we should go backwards. I think we should have less packaged foods and more bulk foods. In my opinion we don't need that many choices on the shelves if we have [organic] products.

Spirituality and Alternative Health

Our discussion of the mimetic impulse is consistent with the emphasis of some on the importance of spirituality as an integral part of alternative health and that which most clearly separates it from biomedicine. The spiritual impulse in alternative health is a renewal of dialogue between self and the world through the inducement of experiential states in which the self is enriched. Contemporary developments in spirituality such as psychic healing, therapeutic touch, guided imagery, meditation, past life regression, crystal healing have roots in the American metaphysical tradition or what Fuller calls "aesthetic Protestantism." What is common to Transcendentalism, nineteenth-century spiritualism, mesmerism, hypnotism, Christian Science, New Thought, is a belief that happiness and physical well-being are consequences of bringing the person into a state of harmony with transpersonal energies and realities.[15] The essential media for access to these energies and realities are objects,, and practices that are in critical ways derived from traditional societies and thought to more closely embody the mimetic impulse.

While an auratic experience can emerge from random encounters, they become more available and more concentrated when the auratic experience is embodied in ritual. For example, drinking Bancha tea alone may or may not suggest other worlds, but drinking the same tea in the ceremonial context of a prelude to a macrobiotic study group may be something else entirely. Fuller describes the way crystals are used ritualistically in healing. Crystals are thought to release healing energies into the body through their stimulation of the body's "spiritual centers" or "chakras," a concept appropriated from Eastern metaphysical traditions.

> Crystal healing is undertaken with the same kind of reverence and mystery as a shamanic ritual. Meticulous attention is given to every stage of preparation. This begins with careful selection of the precise gemstone or crystal that would most enhance one's own personal "vibrations." . . . After the appropriate stone has been selected, the healer must intensify her or his commitment to self-purification. Healers must learn to center themselves inwardly and to purify their psyches or "lower" desires and emotions.[16]

Ritualized healing practices can also be found in more institutionalized settings. At one clinic, to be discussed later, interested patients can go through a week-long "healing intensive" modeled after Native American healing practices such as sweat lodges. Patients go through a wide range of therapies with a mentor or spiritual guide to help them through a process of inner transformation. Of course, spiritualism today as it was in the nineteenth century requires a setting and staging of events under the control of a medium.

The emphasis on spirituality in alternative health should be distinguished from religion. In alternative health the question is the experience of the benevolence of higher powers which guide a person to well-being. Religion, at least to groups in the holistic health network, is criticized because of its moralistic and authoritarian character and the way it strangles life through prohibitions and empty rituals. They want to remove this obstacle to the experience of a vital connection to the world. To say this is to say nothing other than the desire is to reenchant the world.

Among the alternative health networks we studied there is a tension between those who emphasize spirituality as a source of healing and those of a more traditional-religious nature. In the CFC, recommended healing regimes are based largely on natural foods, cleansing, oxidation therapies, and other bodily centered protocols. Good health depends on a systematic treatment of the body through "natural means." Belief in biblical religious principles validates these bodily protocols. They provide their warrant, convincing people of their legitimacy and ultimate efficacy. In the holistic health network, spirituality or a belief in higher benevolent powers is constitutive of healing regimes—meditation, therapeutic touch, biofeedback, guided imagery, past life regression, hypnotism, among others. This does not mean, though, that more bodily centered approaches are neglected in the holistic health network. Instead, both spiritual and bodily protocols are inseparable from one another in holistic health. Interventions such as acupuncture, massage, and herbal medicine are understood in spiritual terms, as vehicles for the opening of the self to deeper realities and powers.

Enchantment is not a moral category but an experiential state that provides an opening to the world and creates happiness and the potential for well-being. As we mentioned earlier, the world becomes a partner in communication and therefore becomes an enlargement of our home. The emphasis on spirituality should be viewed as an expression of the expansion of those areas of life that are removed from moral constraints. The pluralization of forms of life or the multiplication of different conceptions of a good life reflects the growing prominence of questions such as, What do we want to become? What traditions do we want to sustain or discard?, and How should we live? As these questions are asked another set of questions recedes, questions asked in religious traditions and codified in doctrines, even though in certain respects they remain essential: What is the right and wrong way to live? What moral rules should I follow? How do I discipline and restrain myself through moral commands?

In the CFC, there are strong tendencies toward the moralization of illness. Illness, according to many speakers as well as the current leader of the CFC, is a consequence of a deviation from biblical laws. Yet even within this framework erosions of moral absolutism can be discerned. This comes out in the infrequency of discussions of personal culpability for disease. Discussions of strategies to create health and well-being are far more frequent. Health is understood here as it is in the holistic health network, as an increase in energy, vitality, and an enhanced ability to enjoy life. These categories are not moral ones but are essential elements of a view of a "good life." In the holistic health network the demoralization of life is more pronounced and complete. Self-perfection and an increase in energy are uncoupled from any moral perspective. Health and well-being are not consequences of conformity to a moral order but practicing the art of life in the right way. The goal here is to master techniques and practices that make us healthy and happy. In fact, for some spiritually oriented practitioners, the demoralization of health and illness is a precondition for health and well-being.

The following example of a past life regression therapist and one of his clients points to both the demoralization of health and illness and its orientation toward auratic experiences. Ned is a regression therapist who was trained at the Monroe Institute, associated with the ideas and techniques of the mystic Edgar Cayce. He also was trained in hypnotherapy, past life regression, post-traumatic stress therapy, as well as various bodywork techniques such as myofacial release and cranial sacral therapy. He describes his current work as most influenced by Tibetan Buddhism and the belief that "the most important thing to look at is the thought we die with because it locks in all the other karma."

Ned embarked on his career as an alternative health practitioner, like many, as a result of a personal crisis. He and other family members had a number of serious health problems and when his brother was diagnosed with terminal cancer, something told him that he needed to change his life. He "apprenticed" with a healer, "someone who learned everything she knows from dreams and visions," similar to a shaman. This healer taught him "energy medicine" and a way of talking to parts of the body by having a person's consciousness enter that part and talk to the person about its distress. It is this wisdom that comes from the body and speaks from the body that provides the basis for the therapist's interventions. This technique became the basis for much of the work that Ned now does as a regression therapist. He no longer does the hypnotherapy that he learned at the Monroe Institute and instead works directly with his client's complexes as they assume bodily form. While the entry point is often family-centered trauma, Ned may delve into deeper levels of the client's psyche, to traumas that originate in past lives. He now sees his chance meeting with this healer as the "universe presenting me with an opportunity" to serve others.

One of his patients, Sue, who was raised in a fundamentalist household, suffered from depression, anxiety, and chronic pain. She drove for two hours to see Ned after many years of unsuccessful therapy. Her work with Ned began with Ned's observations of the way she held her body and her bodily presence. Ned detected in his observations holding patterns in her "etheric body" a concept derived from the Theosophist mystical tradition. As the sessions continued, Ned stimulated remembrances of past lives and past traumas. Part of the healing experience was for Sue to overcome the guilt and terror from past lives and central to this effort was the work of "spirit guides," "healers," and "teachers" that Ned summoned from other dimensions. The teachers and healers provide guidance to both therapist and patient. A chief lesson learned during this therapy is that there are benevolent entities all around you which if you are open to them will lead you toward health and happiness. The walls that separated her from other people, such as her sister, and from her own body were dismantled. She reported that "she can smell things now around her where before she couldn't. A certain powder that her grandmother wore was present with her." Her headaches lessened and she "is now living more fully in her life."

The journey of this woman is a journey from guilt and neurotic inhibitions to a greater sense of being alive and an ability to experience the pleasures of life in a fuller sense. She is able to reach these higher states through reencountering the world as a partner that suggests directions and new paths. Ned uses techniques derived from Tibetan Buddhism, Theosophy, and bodywork modalities in part derived from Shiatsu and other Eastern settings. Sue's auratic encounter with alternative medicine provides her with a way of relocating her illness and her self in a larger horizon of meaning—the trauma of past lives. After therapy, Sue is not realigned with a moral order but on the contrary is freed from excessive guilt and available for new experiential states.

Diane was trained at the Center for Attitudinal Healing in Washington, D.C., as well as in macrobiotics. She runs a practice where she combines both approaches, nutritional therapy as well as spiritual and psychological counseling. Her philosophy of healing, though, is consistent with the larger spiritual orientation of much of alternative health, emphasizing the connection to a vital source of energy as the path to healing. Diane argues that

> all phenomenon [sic] in this world is energy . . . there's no place where you stop and I start. When you do intuitive diagnosis you can connect with that person. But to do that you have to get yourself together.

Diane does not accept the view that illness is an accident that happens to you. Instead, she encourages her clients to "change their perception of illness" in order to discover what it may teach them about their lives. When a client defines himself by a medical label, Diane knows that this self-definition is part of the problem for it only blocks access to the healing energy, which is available to all of us. In the same vein, Diane understands health as an embodiment of this vital energy, or as she puts it "an appetite for life."

> A healthy person's someone who is adaptable, flexible, who has honest communication and can articulate what they need and (this is a big one) is accepting of other people for who they are unconditionally. Someone who genuinely loves, accepts and respects all of humanity; a good sense of humor and being willing to give to others; a good appetite for life; curiosity and a sense of adventure, and a spirit of gratitude for everything; being a good listener.

Diane's healthy person, like Ned's patient, is available for new experiential states, and is capable of living life to the fullest. Diane does not believe that morality requires obedience to an external authority. Instead, her Catholic upbringing caused "everything to go wrong in my life" because it instilled a pervasive feeling of guilt and fear. Sin, for Diane, is in the mind and can be overcome through a change in one's attitudes and a sense of connection to other people and the wider universe.

The Commodity and the Depletion of Meaning

The distinction between aura and commodity is an important one for us because it sheds light on a crucial tension within alternative health, the tension between its ritualized associations with the past, grounded in bodily practices, and its increasingly commodified character. After all, alternative health services and products are purchased like any other commodity, and alternative health products are becoming a major commercial enterprise. At the same time, for those committed to it, alternative health is much more than this. Alternative health, in other words, exists in this tension between its "auratic" dimension, which gives it a weak utopian character, and its commodified dimension, which helps to integrate it into the larger social order.

Why is it that the commodification of alternative health weakens its utopian and transformative potential? A commodity is an object that is detached from specific uses, rituals, and experiences in order to be exchanged for a price in the market. All commodities share this characteristic and therefore become equivalent to one another in the process of continuous exchange. A work of art in a person's home may have auratic associations that suggest a unique history reexperienced by the owner. On the other hand, for an art dealer that same object is valued only insofar as it can command a high price. In this sense the art object as a commodity is drained of its auratic features. It loses any anchor to a specific world or experience. The commodity abstracts from the lifeworld and serves to disintegrate it. The reference for the commodity is only other commodities in "a continuous mirroring process."[17]

It has been argued that commodities too have their own vapors. They too have references beyond their own use and function. But what is that reference? According to a variety of scholars who have studied advertising, commodities are associated with desired social identities and personal attributes such as popularity, celebrity, authenticity, individuality, all of which are achieved through common purchases.[18] Commodities may also promise a certain kind of pseudo liberation from oppressive styles of life (Virginia Slims, "You've Come a Long Way Baby"). While commodities have vapors, they are not, strictly speaking, auratic. The vapors that surround commodities are consciously constructed images whose purpose is to expand the circle of consumption. In contrast, the associations of an aura are in some sense embedded in the ritualized context within which alternative health products are encountered. These associations interrupt the ongoing homogenization of commodified experience and to some degree impose their meaning on the person. In Benjamin's sense an auratic encounter is like an epiphany. Something fundamental about life flashes before the person and transforms the person's life. What is embedded in the object is a world, or a set of practices that surround the person and provide an orientation and purpose. The person renews meaning actively as she encounters this world and addresses problems within her experience.

Commodities can be reembedded, as well, into daily life. Teenage girls who listen to Madonna and form fan clubs are embedding a constructed image in the pursuit of their own self-definition.[19] But the stability of these definitions, and their staying power, is weak. It is no wonder that postmodernists talk of meaning as deferred, unstable, slippery, the play of empty signifiers. The reference is not to traditions but to lifestyles that are constantly redefined in light of changing definitions of status. An advertised commodity, unlike an object or practice with an aura, has no permanence or unique identity. As Benjamin said, if a commodity could speak it would wish to be in everyone's home and, we would add, only for a brief visit.[20]

The evaporation of the aura with respect to commodities reaches its vanishing point with prescription drugs and their administration. With most commodities there is the promise of a certain status or social position that becomes available through their use—a lifestyle connected to wearing Ralph Lauren clothes. But drugs do not have these suggestions. Instead, drugs are defined within a technical language that cordons them off from the lifeworld.[21] A technical language is most remote from Benjamin's understanding of language as a system of nonsensuous correspondences between the self and the world. A technical language is self-referential and breaks this connection to the lifeworld and the experiences rooted in it. Drugs are not part of social rituals that bind people together and create obligations or memories. When drugs are ingested they disappear into the metabolism of the body. In this sense drugs reinforce biomedicine's world view—a detached physical body operating mechanically and independent of the social norms and practices in the lifeworld.

A typical pharmaceutical drug advertisement illustrates these points. For example, a recent Claritin advertisement is largely taken up with a technical description of its use, contraindications, adverse reactions, and effects of overdoses.[22] The front page of the ad attempts to reconnect the drug to the lifeworld through a picture of a woman staring at the sun pictured in the form of a Claritin tablet. The caption reads, "Nothing but Blue Skies from Now On." However, this effort to recreate a vapor is feeble since it doesn't associate the product with a way of life or position in the world and its promise of well-being is largely neutralized by the technical discussion of side effects that can be found alongside the picture.

The relevance of the analytic distinction we've made between the aura and the commodity is critical to the issue of the coordination of social action as well as identity formation. A commodified experience such as the purchase of a car or an article of clothing is not a source of coordination of actors in the lifeworld. It does not bring people together to pursue common goals. Indeed, commodification isolates people even while they are unified through the act of purchasing.[23] In contrast, auratic experiences are potential sources of action coordination. They provide noninstrumental experiences and therefore extend the realm of sympathy and identification with people and worlds. The aura, in a momentary eruption, bridges the gap between what is near and far, the modern and the premodern. In other words, spatial and temporal distinctions are momentarily overcome and the world becomes unified. For many alternative health patients and prac- titioners, this experience of sympathy and unity is a source for the imagination and an experiential basis for group formation that may have a range of social and political consequences.

Aura, Discourse, and Practice in Two Communities

In the two networks that we've studied, "New Age" (or what we are calling the holistic health network) and Christian, the aura is embedded in alternative health products such as herbs, organic food, and other natural products. This is a source of experiential unity between both groups. For both the aura opens up in an immediate way traditional worlds. The discourse through which they understand and commu- nicate this experience is quite distinct. For most members of HLQ and the co-op, the aura is associated with indigenous groups in Central America, Asia, and to a more limited degree Native Americans in the United States. On the other hand, for the largely conservative Christians in the CFC, the aura is associated with small town and rural American life. In addition there are secondary references to the origins of Christianity in the ancient world. The rural small town associations are consistent with the small town backgrounds of many members of the CFC as well as their ancestors. What blocks access to other traditional worlds are their biblical religious commitments.

A member and activist in the NLG, a vigorous eighty-year-old woman who grows some of her own food and lives in a rural area, described for us her upbringing on a dairy farm in Pennsylvania where she got use to "organic farming" and developed an appreciation for nature, "the fragile web of life" and "the value of self-sufficiency." While describing herself and most CFC members as "conservative Christians" she mixes to some degree holistic health and Christian dis- courses.

> I think of myself as pretty religious—a Presbyterian. Started out as a
> Methodist and married a Congregationalist. We have within us this life
> force and the better we relate to that and to our spiritual well being
> and direction. . . . My husband and I have our devotions. We don't
> do it every day but we certainly do a lot of praying these days for

wisdom and to make the right choices in his healing. . . . You know for thousands of years people had medicine men but they believed in them. And that's how Christ did it. He brought out within the person this belief and probably got their immune systems to make a real quick switch.

While there is a certain eclecticism reflected in these comments, other CFC members' references are more consistent with the biblical tradition. With these members the achievement of health must be grounded in explicit biblical passages. The different discourses have interesting consequences in terms of the practices of both groups. CFC members tend to shy away from the spiritually oriented approaches common in the holistic health network, such as meditation, reiki, past life regression, various forms of mysticism, the use of crystals and shamanism. On the other hand, they embrace a wide range of protocols that directly effect the body and which are at times quite experimental, such as oxidation therapies that involve suffusing the body with ozone or hydrogen peroxide and radical detoxification programs that emphasize cleansing the colon over extended periods of time. The holistic health discourse allows for a degree of openness to a variety of spiritual as well as physical protocols that the Christian discourse precludes because certain spiritual protocols are thought to be demonic and pagan.

Apart from this general distinction, there are more specific ways in which discourse and practice interpenetrate in both groups. In the CFC, discourse works its way through practice in the form of validation of the alternative health protocols people are committed to (it is consistent with biblical teachings). For example, at CFC meetings patient testimonials are common, describing their illness and road to recovery. The protocols they commit themselves to must be "consistent with God's plan for good health." While specific passages of the Bible are rarely mentioned at meetings, such references can be found in some of literature displayed and distributed at meetings. For example one newsletter, called "God's Plan For Good Help (Vol. 2, no. 4)," justifies organic farming and the use of natural foods with specific biblical references.

We need to educate people to get back to God's food and not man's food. When we alter God's food, we bring on disease. God made food with many nutrients. Man has taken those nutrients out. When the nutrients are gone, it becomes a poison to our system . . . [In contrast to white sugar] Honey is mentioned in the Bible as a good food. Proverbs 24:13 states, "My son, eat thou honey, because it is good; and the honeycomb, which is sweet to thy taste." We also alter other foods such as salt. Rock salt, the way God made it, has many minerals in it. Table salt, has one or two minerals. Are we smarter than God? Do we need to take the minerals out? These simple facts must be taught to our people, for God's Word states, "My people are destroyed for lack of knowledge." (Hosea 4:6) God wants His knowledge to be known. Psalm 67:2 states, "For I will restore health unto thee, and I will heal thee of thy wounds, saith the Lord . . ."

Secondly, discourse also encourages people to stay the course through difficult times because it provides a fund of optimism that the protocol will work. One woman, diagnosed with advanced breast cancer and given a few months to live, found the courage to engage in her own healing regime when she came to the realization that she was "in God's hands." As she said, "I prayed to God for help and committed myself to fight." After five weeks of rigorous "detoxification" and nutritional "rejuvenation" she was "cancer free" and wrote a book about her experiences (we will discuss her story in more detail in chapter 4). Another cancer patient, a colleague of ours, went to an alternative cancer clinic when his cancer had progressed to the terminal stage but did not continue the rigorous protocols when he returned home because his religious faith did not give him hope and the courage to continue the demanding course. Finally, the discourse serves to unify members in a common healing community who support and encourage each other. They have a commitment to a common religious tradition embedded in a single text. Sharing a common Christian culture cements bonds of solidarity expressed at the opening prayer in meetings, visits to sick members' homes, among other things.

The spiritual eclecticism of the holistic health network precludes the discourse from functioning as a unifying force and as an external guarantee of the success of the protocol. There is nothing intrinsically Christian about organic farming, natural foods, the use of herbs, oxidation therapies. All of them can be grafted onto a variety of discourses. On the other hand, the eclectic spiritual discourse of the holistic health network resonates in practices that range from mediation, guided imagery, past life regression, shamanism, yoga, Tai Chi, and even to the use of herbs. In this way the discourse of the holistic health network is more constitutive of holistic health practices than in the CFC where protocols are not intrinsically Christian. Ironically, engaging in alternative health protocols may open up Christians to holistic health sensibilities more than the reverse. The eclecticism that is at the heart of alternative health is suffused with holistic health sensibility (an appreciation for pluralism, and for diverse healing practices from around the world), which Christians experience when they become committed to alternative health. The NLG activist quoted earlier illustrates this temptation and pull of Christian alternative health activists toward holistic health orientations.

The Aura and the Recovery of Meaning

Preserving scattered objects, images, and practices rooted in prior worlds, even when promiscuously quoted, is of considerable importance. What is significant is the partial preservation of forms of life that are potential resources for the critique of and resistance to the depletion of meaning in everyday life. These forms of life are appropriated for the purpose of maintaining health or coping with illness. The fact that this appropriation is rooted in the travails of the body gives it a potency not available when we eat at a Chinese restaurant, visit a Native American art gallery, or buy hand made goods at a Guatemalan craft store. No one can claim that eating Chinese food provides a basis for transforming one's life and distancing oneself from dominant institutions and practices. In contrast, alternative health's practices, since they are integral to maintaining or seeking health, frequently do have life transforming significance since health and illness are so closely bound up with who we are and how we live.

Rebecca, a nurse who practices therapeutic touch at a major hospital, describes herself this way,

> I am what one priest called a cafeteria Catholic. I just take what I want and leave the rest. But I am a Theosophist. I am an . . . I definitely, I mean, I do yoga, I do Tai Chi, I have a Buddha sitting in my . . . by my pond, and I have a garden with a Virgin Mary in it. So if you come to my house you see everything. You see American Indian things, you see . . . definitely, you know, focused on the Chuna Way. I definitely believe in the cycles of life and reincarnation. . . .

This quotation of the past is central to how Rebecca lives and has provided the basis for her professional work where she combines a variety of ancient healing traditions in a hospital setting.

Eileen, the co-op staff member introduced earlier, also says that she experimented with "many different diets, health regimes, affirmation schemes . . . [in search of a cure for her illness]. When I started out looking for answers I would almost follow anything that came along." Eventually she found an answer in Eastern spiritual practices. But, she thinks of this as part of a larger dialogue with different healing traditions. Eileen's commitments to healing practices rooted in other cultures transformed her life and gave her back her health. This led her to a commitment to working in the co-op and introducing customers to her experiences with traditional healing practices. As we mentioned earlier, when we talked to her she was disappointed with the direction of the co-op and the nature of her work within it. She was concerned that the co-op was turning into a supermarket and she was a mere worker in it, helping to sell its products.

Another example of how the quotation of the past has life-transforming potential comes from our participation in a macrobiotic study group. Macrobiotic cooking is a Japanese-derived food regime that requires significant time for food preparation. Precisely because this dietary regime requires participants to cook at certain temperatures, combine foods in certain ways, eat foods only in certain seasons, its mastery cannot be learned casually but only through conscious study, often times in study groups. Agnes, a twenty-eight-year-old woman who had chronic health problems, found relief through a regimen that consisting principally of a macrobiotic diet. She told us that she enjoys cooking because it slows down time and evokes latent meanings connected to nature and seasonal change. In fact her emergence in the world of macrobiotics has served to enchant her life. For example, when Agnes gets sick she believes that "the universe is telling me to slow down." Because of her habit of denying her emotions through frenetic activity, illness, she believes, contains a message that speaks to her and provides a chance for her to transform her life. Though she has suffered from cancer and alcoholism, the world once again is livable for her.

The practice of macrobiotics leads others to move from concern about health on an individual level to engage in a "diagnosis for our times." Another member of the macrobiotic study group, Bobbi, told us,

> I think that the way we eat is a huge problem that has an effect on the environment and the family structure as well . . . um, you know, people don't have time to eat well because nobody's home to cook.

Fast food is a way of life for American people and I think that that's really . . . it contributes to poor physical and mental health, poor family relations. You grab a Happy Meal at McDonald's. I don't think that does as much for a person's inside-out, you know in their head, in their body . . . it just doesn't do it.

Here we see that the slowing down of time, and the heightened sensitivity to nature in macrobiotics provides the resources for some to critically distance themselves from the unexamined routines of everyday life.

A number of acupuncturists told us that their approach to healing releases and reorganizes "energy," which is understood through frameworks borrowed from Chinese metaphysical systems. John, who works part time in a practice with a chiropractor and a naturopath, was trained in "traditional acupuncture" in England with a doctor who "focuses on the acupuncture that was lost during the Cultural Revolution." He has done past life regression to help him come to terms with his relationship with his parents and believes in a "multidimensional self." He is interested in Chinese herbology. He was heavily involved in the sixties counterculture and for a short period helped his fiancé run a natural food restaurant. Shortly after his marriage he and his wife traveled to South America where he "became opened to the diversity of beliefs about healing." He realized that "there is more to life that what meets the eye and more than I suspected growing up in a [small town]." His view of acupuncture is that it addresses the spirit as well as the body. When he inserts a needle it "hits various levels—physical, emotional, and spiritual." He can tell if the patient is experiencing a spiritual problem by "determining what level the Chi is reached." He looks for places where the Chi is blocked. The opening session is devoted to a two-hour consultation where John sees himself as a facilitator or guide "exploring unexamined dimensions" of the client. John believes that "we live in a yang society, a driven society . . . where we have a drive to control." This stems from the Cartesian separation of mind from body and since "women are associated with the body we have to control women." He disapproves of the fitness movement that tells us "that we have to work our bodies so that they become fit and don't give us trouble as opposed to working with, co-creating with nature."

Allison is a massage therapist who is active in HLQ and has served on the HLQ board of directors for a number of years. Allison got interested in massage as a result of a personal crisis. After completing her degree in a top tier university (in English), Allison worked for a short period in a health food store. "I started learning about nutrition and food and that sort of led into a whole investigation of plants and their properties and that bridged into herbs a little bit and all that sort of thing." But Allison wanted to do something with her expensive education and soon found herself working as a copy editor and legal coordinator for an advertising agency. She realized after a period of time that it was "nearly an impossible task" to ensure that the advertising coming out of the agency was "true and legal," which was her job. Moreover, she disliked the routine, "tracing the same path to the office and going up the elevator every day, and being in the same cubicle."

Allison now realizes that she responded to this crisis in her life by becoming sick. She contracted mononucleosis and when she returned to work she had "debilitating pain throughout her body. I couldn't move without throwing up. I could barely see light." After numerous tests, her doctors couldn't tell what was wrong, "so I had to find a way to make that meaningful for myself." Upon being released from the hospital she sought help from alternative practitioners, exploring in greater depth some of the healing traditions she dabbled in when she worked in the natural foods store. When she regained her health, Allison realized that "I had not explored all my gifts. I had spent this time developing my intellect but perhaps I had other gifts along with my intellect." She now sees her illness as a message to change her life. Her illness interrupted the progress of her life and gave her an opportunity to reassess its direction. Her experience working in the natural food store in exploring natural foods, herbs, and alternative dietary regimes provided cultural resources, connections to diverse traditions that she called upon later.

In Allison's practice as a massage therapist she sees clients with work-related muscle problems and pain, clients who are referred to her from psychologists (often gestalt therapists), clients with back pain that may stem from a death, divorce, or significant emotional loss, and clients whose pain stems from a fall or accident and the resulting trauma. Her therapeutic approach requires that she understand the client's lifeworld, the connection between the client's pain or discomfort and his work, emotional life, and social relationships.

In all three cases, with macrobiotics, acupuncture, and massage therapy, the instrumental character of food preparation and bodily healing is contested. Advocates of macrobiotics are sustaining a practice that contests the speeding up of food preparation and consumption in the form of meals that are deritualized and devoid of meaning (eating on the run in order to fill up). The abstraction of time from specific context, its homogenization, and the way activities are accelerated through the managerial use of time are contested (schedules, appointments, meetings). Massage therapists and practitioners of traditional acupuncture relate bodily pain to practices and issues in the lifeworld of the person, such as posture, emotional distress, type of shoes, and work habits around the home, exercise routines. These are not just physical or anatomical issues but relate to a person's unique way of life. In this sense the body is not just a physical system identical to every other but a penumbra of specific meanings.

Peggy, who works part time now as a college instructor in the health sciences, began what she describes as her "accidental spiritual journey" when her baby died of congenital heart failure at four months old. She had a "panic attack" during her seventh month and her doctor prescribed Valium for her. After the death of her baby she continued to take Valium, Zanax, and sleeping medications to cope with her stress, anxiety, and grief. Her health deteriorated shortly after with recurring stomach problems, sleeplessness, and anxiety. She felt she was "out of control." Around this time, Peggy saw a sign for a meditation class that began this "accidental spiritual journey."

Along with her meditation classes, she sought help from a macrobiotic counselor and a homeopathic physician. Both suggested a change in her diet that soon led to an improvement in her condition. Her homeopathic physician also recommended that she take a yoga class and she became "intrigued by back flower remedies." Now she has decided to cut back on her hours at work in order to appreciate what is valuable about her life. As she looks back on her experiences she believes that her obstetrician should not have prescribed Valium for her and that her stomach problems were misdiagnosed. As Peggy puts it, "The male medical profession is so male-oriented and has so often missed the boat. They just forgot the whole aspect of caring. And maybe I think that women are more nurturing, more healing oriented." In addition to a budding feminist consciousness, her immersion in other healing and spiritual traditions has led to an interest in the Hospice movement and in "viewing death as an opportunity for enlightenment." She has also become a critic of the commodified world around her and is especially critical of how commercials on TV "sets how we're supposed to live, how women should look, dress, be, act, how they should treat their families." Here's a snippet of her story in her own words.

I strive for a macrobiotic approach. While I have not given up meat, I have added grains. I've obviously stayed off dairy. I've added more vegetables. I'm just more interested in that whole realm of nutritional practice. I still practice homeopathy. I practice bach flower remedies, they deal with emotional issues. I do yoga. Probably the most substantial change in my life has to do with meditation, and I do practice meditation every day. I think a lot of it comes back to that. From that, not only do I continue having interest in things that are more kind to the body, there are lots of other things that it has spawned interest in for me. It's directly related now to my interest in Buddhism. I'm not at all the person that I was even a year ago; I'm much more low key. I'm in a very odd place, a strange sort of place, a figuring out what it is that I want to be and what I'm doing with myself from a professional perspective. But when I directed a medical records department I worked very hard, very long hours, and I think that the stress was directly the cause of a great deal of my health problems. And I felt helpless, I felt that there wasn't a damn thing I could do about that, that's just how life is and you just have to cope and it's amusing to watch TV because commercials for various medications and acid relievers, they make it look just like that's the way it has to be, you have to live a fast-paced life, you have to eat junky foods, and you have to run for twenty-four hours a day. I feel like I'm waking up for the first time in my life in the last year; I'm looking at all those things. I've cut back in my work; I'm more of a part-time basis now. Things are very different for me. And all this is very much connected, there is not one thing that I can pull out of there as being a root cause.

For Peggy, Allison, and John, the distancing that is made possible through the quotation of the past provides a resource for critical reflection about themselves and the world around them. In other words, these quotations of the past are an experiential basis for the critique of elements of modern life.

The Commodification of the Past

While alternative health practices and products have auratic suggestions that have the capacity to change people's lives within certain limits, these suggestions are not without their tensions and contradictions. When removed from a ritualized context their capacity to shape lives seems limited. Why is this so? When the past is made available through fragments that are placed next to each other in a supermarket format their impact is muted. The danger is that the quotation of the past may only be filtered through the commodity form. What is the experiential content of encountering the fragments of "thirty" traditions side by side on a supermarket or health store shelf? The undifferentiated unity with prior worlds is largely filtered or weakened. In this sense, this is an instance of the rationalization of the aura. Instead of an object looking back at you, here there is only a glance. What gives the aura its life-transforming potential is its connection to the travails of the body and the ritualized contexts of their use.

The food co-op in Pittsburgh is a place where organic food can be purchased, and it is owned co-operatively. But in addition, the co-op has a unique identity that differentiates it from the grocery store. Customers and staff can be found in overalls, old tee shirts, and jeans, clothes that suggest indigenous and rural lifeworlds. There are also some unique products such as organic fruits and vegetables, alternative supplements, and reading material ranging from astrology of the ancient Mayans to vegetarian cookbooks and handicrafts. Even the lack of efficiency, for example, long waits at the checkout counter because of long personal discussions between customers and staff, reduces the sense that it's simply a business. But these associations are somewhat ephemeral and superficial. After all the organic vegetables and supplements are marketed like any other commodity in which the past becomes a quotation rather than a reenactment. A person can wear a Peruvian coat, buy a package of Chinese herbal tea, order a glass of carrot juice, which suggests a preindustrial encounter with food, and then drive away in their Volvo to their suburban home.

Moreover, an examination of the history of food co-ops illustrates the tension between commodification and a politicized reappropriation of the past. During the early 1970s co-ops were most distant from the commodified supermarket model of food distribution. Instead of displaying a variety of packaged, prepriced food items, consumers would choose from bulk items in brown bags, which had to be weighed and marked with a price. Attached to some items were descriptions of the worlds from which they were lifted and the political struggles that were going on there. Customers checked themselves out and there were no paid staff members, only volunteers.[24] A long-time co-op staff member in the Pittsburgh co-op whom we interviewed lamented this shift from the earlier model toward the co-op becoming "just another supermarket with an array of packaged items for sale." Nevertheless, the co-op still carries bulk items and has retained handwritten descriptions of some items like organic coffee and the nonprofit networks in which they are embedded. The volunteer concept also remains to some degree with the use of "skill workers" who volunteer their services in return for a discount on the food they purchase.

At one Wellness 2000 awards banquet there were a variety of rituals and activities including drumming, holding hands in a circle and engaging in meditation, and a performance of Native American dance, suggesting Native American and Eastern religious practices. Participants greeted one another with an air of conviviality and informality, hinting at the friendliness of small town life. When meals were served a variety of organic vegetarian dishes suggested ancient modes of farming. Yet, the familiarity tended to be superficial, and the combining of various traditions seemed discordant and inauthentic—foreign to the social roots of many of the participants. The collection of rituals from diverse sources had to be planned and administered, a kind of constructed naturalness, limiting their experiential impact. Overall, what was involved was not a form of life but a display of "ruins" from many divergent ones. In contrast to Benjamin who always saw a ruin from a dialectical perspective, holding the unity of catastrophe and redemption within its form, here only a romanticized view of the past is evoked. The suffering and injustices that are embedded in traditional worlds are erased. Adorno and later Benjamin warned of the danger of an uncritical celebration of the past because of its connection to regressive and even fascistic political movements.[25]

Lives unfold in the tension between the aura and the commodity, between the fleeting encounter with traditional worlds that have critical potential and the deritualized practices of consumer culture. Rebecca, the nurse who practices therapeutic touch at a major hospital, illustrates some of the tensions in trying to combine ancient healing traditions and their auratic qualities with biomedicine. Her practice at a major hospital pulls her in contradictory directions. On the one hand, Rebecca has mastered traditional healing practices that she tries to integrate into her work with patients. But on the other hand, institutional pressures pull her in a different direction. The commercial setting of the hospital creates pressures to spend less time with patients to become more cost effective. In addition she is under pressure to conform to the allopathic model and marginalize her identity as a shamanic healer, trained in a Polynesian healing tradition. For example, in her practice she draws upon ancient healing traditions that "have been around for a very long time and so there's some truth in it and we draw upon that." But when she tries to incorporate this wisdom in her work, she has to translate the metaphysical language, such as "prana" and "chakras," into a physicalist language that is comprehensible to the biomedical system. This translation results in an inevitable loss of meaning. Terms such as *prana* and *chi* suggest design and purpose in nature to which we can gain access and to some degree communicate with through ritualized practices. On the other hand, when these terms are translated into "energy fields" what is lost is the sense of nature's mystery and purpose and the traditions which these forces evoke.

It's not only the discourse that is thrown into tension in the hospital setting but the practices themselves. Rebecca argues that her practice is totally consistent with biomedicine and her institutional setting. Yet when it came to discussing actual cases she revealed problems with her ability to practice her craft because of the overmedication of patients and what she calls the intolerance of medical professionals concerning her work.

One alternative health care practitioner who has spoken at the CFC and who publishes a monthly newsletter on health refers both to biblical passages and traditional methods of growing food and botanical medicine, justifying the latter in terms of biblical teachings. Here the evocation of the aura is explicitly grounded in religious teachings, mostly Christian but at times from eclectic spiritual sources. At the same time, in this newsletter, a line of products are advertised and promoted with an underlying philosophy resembling Dale Carnegie's *Power of Positive Thinking*. Readers are instructed in how to become effective distributors of products and how to be financially independent and successful.

This same tension between the aura and the commodity is present in the popular literature on alternative health. One instance is an autobiographical account of a medical doctor, Lewis Mehl-Madrona, who tries to mediate between the medical model and the monetary pressures of the health care industry and his own native healing traditions.[26] In the course of his residency Dr. Madrona became disenchanted with the lack of care and concern for individual patients, from the technological model of birth employed in maternity wards to examples of iatrogenesis and unnecessary surgery and their concealment. This vague dissatisfaction with the allopathic model encouraged him to rediscover his Native American roots and their relevance for the care and healing of sick people. This happened in the course of a crisis in his professional life, which compelled him to rethink why he was in medicine and how he wanted to practice it.

Eventually he had a vision or dream in which his ancestors spoke to him as spiritual guides to lead him to a new direction in his life. This happened during a sweat lodge ceremony, which opened him up to this metaphysical experience. The notion of invoking spirits as sources of guidance is now central to his medical practice.

Dr. Madrona's selective appropriation of his own past led him to reembed medicine in a larger horizon of meaning. Dr. Madrona now occupies a position at a major hospital where he combines elements of the allopathic model in an uneasy tension with alternative approaches. As we will discover later, Dr. Madrona's commitment to Native American healing traditions caused him considerable trouble in his professional life, which he continues to cope with as best he can.

Orientations toward the Past

The ruins of the past appropriated by alternative health allow us to reflect upon the larger question of the relation between modernity and tradition. A ruin, by its fragmentary nature, suggests the potential to assemble these fragments into new combinations. In this way the ruin becomes consistent with the modern notion of agency. We, human beings, must put the fragments of the past together in order to reinvent the world around us. Ironically, this potential for agency embedded in ruins is made possible by the forces of global capitalism and its rampant commodification across the expanse of time and space. Benjamin understood this when he argued that the commodified form of the ruin lifts it from its mythological and cultic contexts and allows it to have a redemptive promise. But on the other hand the commodified form of this separation threatens to erase its redemptive charge.

In this spirit, a distinction can be made between actors who self-consciously understand their stance as assemblers of fragments of prior worlds and those who are not aware of the creative and reinvented nature of their appropriation of the past. Instead, they imagine that they can escape the fragmented character of traditions and put one emphatic past back together again. On this basis we can make a distinction between the character of different social movements. The question is, Do we belong to multiple, reinvented communities or an organic community that can be holistically revived?

These distinct ways of appropriating the past can illuminate certain aspects of the two alternative health networks we've been studying. The playful and promiscuous appropriation of tradition fragments characterizes the holistic health network. On the other hand, participants in the CFC and NLG seek to recover a traditional way of living rooted in small town and rural American life, values that more fully embody biblical principles. Not only do most of the members of the CFC and NLG come from small town backgrounds but their notion of a good and healthy life rotates around traditional farming with its emphasis on monoculture, monocrops, and the biblical idea of leaving the land fallow every seven years so the soil does not become devitalized. This evocation of the past is not understood as something that is constructed but is imposed upon them by their religious dogma. Their educational and class background makes it less likely that they will have had experiences in other countries and with diverse cultures.

Despite these different tendencies, there are counterinfluences that grow out of the commonality of their commitment to alternative health practices. To the extent to which CFC participants engage in a wide range of alternative health practices, they will be exposed to tradition fragments that will relativize the authority of one emphatic past. In other words, they will be surrounded by a variety of auras that will weaken their exclusively biblical focus. Among the CFC participants we interviewed there is a self-conscious drive to anchor alternative health in biblical sources but the breath of alternative health punches holes in their conceptual framework,which makes it difficult for them to formulate what they are doing without slippage. One NLG activist in the context of discussing her millennial beliefs saw Christ as a healer because he could engage in techniques to trigger effective immune responses. The language of the "immune system" and the understanding of how it works come from a wide selection of alternative health care literature, which includes references to Eastern metaphysical traditions.

The following table, which develops distinctions made in this chapter, is a beginning of an attempt to think through the larger question of the way the past enters into the orientation of actors as they seek to transform the world around them. One orientation involves an effort to renew a single tradition that provides the key to redemption. Many ethnic-nationalist movements illustrate this orientation. A broader way to think about these movements is provided by Barrington Moore who argued that "conservative movements" (and their extreme embodiment in fascism) throughout Western history have had the following characteristics.[27] These movements seek "thoroughgoing moral regeneration" in the absence of any analysis of the social forces that threaten their interest. They evoke images of life

Table 3.1   Modes of Appropriation of the Past in Social Movements

	Messianic Impulse	
	Weak	Strong
Dialectical	Postmodern movements (Zapatistas)	Revolutionary Socialist Movements (German S. P. D. in the 1920s and I. W. W.)
Undialectical	"New Social Movements" (radical feminism, deep ecology, hippies, alternative health)	Millenarian and ethnic nationalist movements (Islamic fundamentalism)

Explanation of Terms

Dialectical—reflective appropriation of the past which maintains an awareness of gains and losses, costs and achievements of modernity.

Undialectical—affirms uncritically a romanticized view of the past as a solution to the cost of modernity.

Strong messianic impulse—a strong sense that the world will be redeemed or emancipated through some collective agent.

Weak messianic impulse—a vague sense of a better world suggested in images and practices without a conception of a collective agent.

as an organic whole connected to the soil through which they seek warm and secure relationships to the cold and impersonal pressures of urban cosmopolitan life. These conservative movements do not justify their assertions through arguments that can be debated and revised. Instead, the model of the past that they celebrate is dogmatically affirmed. We characterize these movements as "undialectical" in that their affirmation of themselves and their own traditions is uncritical and wholly affirmative. In addition, the affirmation of the future as renewal of the past is explicitly put forth in arguments (regardless of their simplicity), hence our designation "strong messianic impulse." This "regressive utopianism," to use Melucci's formulation, amounts to "the reduction of reality to one all-embracing principle." These movements, many of which have a religious dimension, may well be gaining ground as a mode of resistance to the hegemony of global capitalism.[28]

Revolutionary movements, as Wolf argued, attempt to renew elements of the past (the values and connections embedded in village life) as the model for the transformed future, but, unlike conservative movements, do not forget the stagnation and oppression in traditional life.[29] The agent for the renewal is the working class and other class fractions while for conservative movements the agent is the "people" identified in ethnic or nationalist terms.

A third orientation involves a weak but dialectical appropriation of tradition. Evan's discussion of the Zapatista movement in Chiapias embodies this position.[30] Zapatistas refer to their vision of the future in poetic metaphors; "a whisper of a new world, so new that it is but an intuition in the collective heart." This suggests a better world that is only hinted at and not systematically developed. But this whisper is not a promissory note without complication. The Zapatistas affirm democratic decisionmaking and the rights of women thereby criticizing the elements of their own traditional past even while affirming their solidarity, self-sufficiency, and organic ties to the natural world, which the past whispers to them. There is, in other words, "a mutual subversion of the traditional and the modern."[31]

The alternative health movement illustrates the final orientation to the past. Here the past is evoked in flickering images of reconciliation with the natural world. These flickering images sustain hope for a unspecified and untheoretically worked through desire for a different world. Unlike the Zapatistas, though, there is no recognition of the oppression and barbarism that are embedded in these whispers and images form the past. The images are simply celebrated.

The reference to the soil in Barrington Moore's characterization of conservative movements, alternative health's conception of the organic as an equivalent to the traditional, and the Zapatistas commitment to agricultural self-sufficiency suggest an extension to the meaning of the word tradition. In modern social movements references to nature increasingly become entangled with or replace references to tradition. Nature and tradition become interchangeable signifiers because for modern men and women it becomes increasingly difficult to renew tradition in some unmediated sense. What "Nature" provides is a way of distancing ourselves from the driving force of instrumental rationality and commodification. As Melucci says, "nature appears as that which resists external pressures because it lies beyond instrumental rationality. It has the inestimable weight of a 'given entity' in opposition to the enforced 'socialization' of identity by the new forms of domination."[32] For Melucci, one feature of new social movements is their appeal to nature as a basis for resistance to systems of control that extend outward through the globe and inward to biological processes.[33]

Why is the undialectical celebration of the past in alternative health not a source of regressive tendencies as is the case with conservative movements, for instance, ethnic-nationalist movements? The answer is that the past is selectively quoted in the form of the auras that surround products, rituals, and healing regimes. The past is not transformed into a program but into expectations, whispers, and intimations that weakly suffuse alternative health care practices. In contrast, the popularity of organic food and natural health remedies in Nazi Germany shows how a valorization of nature was incorporated into fascist ideology.[34] Anti-urbanism and the notion that land is a source of national unity, the association of physical health with national revitalization, and a critique of bourgeois decadence were all part of the fascist revulsion at elements of modernity in the name of a revitalized national identity.[35] Ironically, the commodification of alternative health throughout the United States and Western Europe makes this kind of essentialist deployment of the natural less likely.

The chief danger of alternative health's "weak messianic impulse" is not that it will give rise to reactionary political movements but that its impulse for change will be eliminated through commodification. As we have argued, commodification erases auratic associations with the past and displaces them with associations constructed by advertising agencies to expand market transactions. In addition, commodification is closely entwined with the compartmentalization of everyday life. One can shop at a conventional supermarket as well as a co-op, ingest pharmaceutical drugs along with herbs, meditate and work fifty hours a week. In other words, the auratic encounter with the past in alternative health is threatened because it's interwoven with encounters and commitments to work, consumption as well as physical structures such as shopping malls, suburbs, and automobiles that are hegemonic. The failure to appreciate these compromises can lead to an overinflated view of a person's independence from dominant institutions. In this view, individuals have the power through changing consciousness and health practices (becoming more natural) to achieve complete immunity from the core institutions of modern society.

In summary, the contradictions of alternative health are most clearly expressed in their valorization of the "natural."[36] The natural suggests traditional worlds that people long to enter for happiness and meaning. This yearning expresses a mimetic drive for unity and roots, for a noninstrumental experience through which people can find a home. It can be the vehicle for the hope of redemption. But, if appropriated in an uncritical and uncompromised way, the natural can have ideological uses by freezing the imagination and thwarting the drive for human freedom and emancipation. In alternative health, the natural and the past are both good, without complications or contradictions. This naiveté is not ironic or playful, characteristic of the postmodern sensibility. What is not appreciated in alternative health is how the invocation of tradition is also a repetition of catastrophe as well as redemption, a dialectical point that Benjamin emphasized.

The tendency to blame individuals for their ill health, to neglect the social sources of illness, and to turn good health into an all-encompassing world view are tendencies within alternative health that flow from its uncritical appropriation of "the natural." However, the weak character of alternative health's appropriation of tradition reduces this danger. Unlike conservative movements and fascism, no one tradition is associated with nature and healthy living. Moreover, the commodification of alternative health products and services prevents any particular sense of "the natural" from providing a source of purpose and direction. In short, the alternative health movement must navigate between the twin dangers of too much meaning and not enough.

In light of these compromises, what happens to the capacity of people to locate and orient themselves when traditions are appropriated through quotation? The self-understanding of actors becomes fragmented in the sense that the past is not integrated into a comprehensive system of meaning. In other words, the past is not the basis for a coherent world view. Yet, the selective identification with the past provides a weak source of meaning. It suggests practices, values, associations that shape and give meaning to lives. Unlike the way commercial products invoke the past, in alternative health products are linked to a form of life that involves ongoing practices and commitments.

We have found in Walter Benjamin's argument that the search for meaning does not enfold in time but interrupts it a relevant resource for conceptualizing a fundamental drive in alternative health. Alternative health interrupts the flow of time through its invocation of the natural and its auratic connections to traditional worlds. The invocation of traditional worlds is essentially contentless. It is more like a yearning, a series of vague and unspecified hopes and comforting associations. A world is invoked but not occupied. Perhaps the weak messianic impulse evokes utopian yearnings but without the dangers of regressive tendencies implicated in an unqualified valorization of the archaic. Utopia is cut down to size and contained in the identification with small things.

What mediates the connection between the enchantment of nature and the weak suffusion of utopia into social movements is how enchantment works on the individual, transforms her, and makes her available for new kinds of social and political interactions. We call, following Foucault, this process of self-transformation, the "care of the self," which in our words is the way enchantment becomes instantiated through bodily practices. In the next chapter we will explore the meaning of the "care of the self" and how alternative health regimes open people to wider social and political commitments.

CHAPTER 4

Technologies of the Self

In the last chapter we explored how alternative health products and practices enchant nature and release the semantic energies that were once preserved in myth and religious ritual. It does this, however, in a quotational form that reduces, while not eliminating, its reactionary and antimodern potential. In alternative health there is no one comprehensive version of the past that is the standard to criticize the present and to pursue in the future. Instead, the past takes the form of fragments that evoke images of reconciliation with the world.

In this chapter we explore the alternative health regime or what we call, in the spirit of Foucault, technologies of the self. By and large, people who are engaged in these regimes suffer from chronic illness. This means that their illnesses are not amenable to a quick cure through the interventions of conventional medicine, often creating a series of frustrating encounters with medical expertise.[1] The devotion of people in alternative health to regimes of self-care should not be confused with the notion of "self-care" which is used widely in biomedicine. Instead, a regime is a set of continuous practices based upon principles that are individually tailored depending upon the situation of the person. There is a distinct set of protocols that requires effort and understanding. But the way individuals specifically incorporate these protocols into the texture of their lives is artful. The person must "listen to his/her body" and make decisions, alterations, and adjustments based on situational factors. Since the nature and level of toxicity varies, as does the person's ability to maintain the practice, the person through trial and error must modify the regimes.

The mastery of these regimes is a process of reskilling or the increase of individual competence. As a person begins to use colonics, fasting of various kinds, herbal cleanses, or nutritional regimes, they must be self-conscious about how their body responds. We were told by some of the people we interviewed in the CFC that a "healing crisis" is one common consequence of following an alternative health regime. A "healing crisis" is an apparent worsening of symptoms that results from the application of the regime. What is thought to happen is a weakening of the underlying condition that is the basis for future rejuvenation. How the healing crisis will manifest itself and in what form is impossible to determine beforehand. If a person is not able to interpret the apparent worsening of symptoms as a healing crisis it may precipitate a panic reaction. The panic reaction may lead to terminating the regime. As the person continues the regime in full awareness of his body's responses his competence grows by "doing the work." Competence expands as the person moves into the process of rejuvenation. Here the goal is to experience a state of perfect health.

We focus in this chapter on chronically ill patients, most of whom are members of the CFC and NLG. Ed, CFC's current director, has devoted considerable time to developing his water purification system and on compiling numerous videotapes on the value of various alternative health regimes. These videotapes are shown prior to the opening lecture, where Ed can be found near a table providing information on his water purification invention. His wife Sandra is at another table representing the local food co-op where she works. There one can find information about organic produce as well as various products, sold by the co-op, that are commonly used in an alternative regime. After an opening prayer, people are reminded that while faith is important, passivity in the face of illness is not what God demands. Instead, biblical principles are to guide us in "taking charge of our health" though daily regimes. The precise character of an appropriate health regime is up to each person and depends on a variety of factors, which cannot, we are told, be specified in advance, like a cookbook recipe.

Meetings center around providing information to patients and their families about various alternative health therapies and treatment regimes. In the question and answer session following the lecture, patients often discuss at some length their own experiences with self-care often involving considerable trial and error. Many of the people who attend CFC's monthly meetings can also be found at the many lectures of Maureen Solomon, an alternative health entrepreneur who counsels people with chronic health problems, as well as lectures by practitioners and physicians who practice at cancer clinics in other countries where alternative treatments are used. At these gatherings people do more than listen. They are also meeting places where people share information on their health regimes, support one another, exchange testimonials during question and answer sessions, and gain confidence in their efforts to pursue a path to health, largely independent of conventional medicine.[2] What brings people to these meetings with urgency and commitment is a desire to share their stories about the failure of biomedicine and learn about alternative treatments that will then be woven into their own approach to self-care. In this chapter we rely not only on the accounts of people we have interviewed concerning their regimes but also these more public testimonials.

Eileen, who works in the food co-op, talks about her life in terms of the regimes she explored to cope with her chronic illnesses. For Eileen, life is a project that has to be systematically worked on, and through her explorations of meditation, yoga, cleansing, and alternative nutritional regimes, among others, she transformed herself almost like a work of art. When we interviewed Susan in her home, an elderly NLG activist, she had prepared an eight-page single-spaced account of her life organized around her explorations of different alternative health regimes, which were introduced to her in health spas and clinics. Susan seemed to be in search of some state of perfection, where her body would be returned to a natural state, in harmony with the nature around her. She believes that people have lost the "life skills" that allow them to care for their bodies and their health. For both Eileen and Susan, the health regime is a process of acquiring the skills of taking care of oneself, skills that led both to a critical stance toward medical authority and to other elements of modern societies. These and other stories convinced us that we couldn't understand the micro politics of alternative health unless we examine the alternative health regime. Moreover, these regimes have a significant aesthetic dimension that distances participants from medical supervision since the regime is a unique and artful creation of each patient.

We conceptualize alternative health regimes as aesthetic practices whose goal is the creation of the perfect body in complete harmony with nature. We use the term *aesthetic practice* to refer not simply to the creation of objects by a specialized group of practitioners (artists) but also to practices that ordinary people engage in for the purpose of transforming their lives. This conception of aesthetics and everyday life contests common assumptions about aesthetic practice that tend to split aesthetics into a specialized and autonomous sphere. In contrast, we define "aesthetic practice" as working on the self with skill and stamina for the purpose of achieving self-perfection. Aesthetic practices, we argue, are a source of participation in public life in addition to the more commonly discussed utilitarian[3] and moral sources.[4] Alternative health regimes contain an aesthetic core, a quest for perfect harmony and balance, that step by step makes people available for participation in public life. In this way, as we will demonstrate, the body is recovered as a source of opposition and social transformation.[5]

Our analysis of the aesthetic dimension of alternative health regimes is stimulated by a theme in Michel Foucault's later writings.[6] As is well known, Foucault attempted to answer some of the problems connected with his totalizing critique of power and knowledge regimes. In the classical notion, power was a force of repression. It squeezed and destroyed elements that were distinct from it and therefore evoked opposition. Power was not total because it implied that resistance could be rationally grounded in terms of normative claims. Foucault argued that power was productive. It formed the very reality it suffused. Therefore, there was nothing outside the power/knowledge regimes except its own workings and discursive justifications. But Foucault's critics argued that this notion of power denied any critical standpoint or perspective that could contest power.[7] Foucault himself appeared to agree with this position since he refused to identify the source of resistance to power/knowledge regimes in reason or in some version of desire or *"lebensphilosophie."* In Foucault's words, "we should be able to discover the things themselves in their primordial vitality," but he argues that this is not possible.[8]

Despite this rejection, the emphasis in Foucault's work points to a partiality for those who are crushed by power—the insane, the imprisoned, and sexual deviants. Yet Foucault cannot provide a normative foundation for this position. As a way of conceiving of an exit from the totalizing grip of power, Foucault began to explore "technologies of the self" that were in some sense autonomous from power regimes as well as self-directed.[9] By technologies of the self, Foucault meant sets of practices that can be mastered in order to produce a new human being. He found embedded in ancient Greek and Roman sexual practices expressions of this process of self-mastery. These practices were not concerned with self-exploration, confessions, or the disclosure of secrets, requiring endless talk under the supervision of experts. Neither did such practices involve the application of abstract rules that fit everyone. Instead, these technologies had no psychological depth, but they did produce certain kinds of human beings. The cultivation of voice, clothing, gestures, manner of walking, or regimes to intensify desire through self-mastery create beauty in unique ways in a person's life. In this way, Foucault claims, the power connected to self-mastery and self-perfection became synonymous with liberation and therefore distinct from power/knowledge regimes. What is liberating about this, according to Foucault, is that these explorations are uniquely created and therefore cannot be codified and subjected to bureaucratic supervision.

With Foucault, we agree that there is an aesthetic escape from the grip of power regimes in the form of what he calls technologies of the self. But we redefine aesthetics in a way that critically departs from Foucault and more generally from postmodernism. In addition, unlike Foucault's work where the body is an effect of discipline and power, we see the body as a resource that points people toward the path of resistance.

The Aesthetic Project of Alternative Health Regimes

What are the principles of alternative health regimes? In much of alternative medicine, good health requires the removal of toxicity from the body. There are various protocols through which toxic material is removed from the body. Cleansing and fasting programs are central—involving herbs, enemas, colonics, mineral and vitamin supplements, and juicing, among other things. One elderly woman, an active member of the Natural Living Group, told us about a detoxification experience she had involving fasting at an alternative health clinic:

> And then just before we left, some of the other guests and I were talking about dry fasting so we thought we would try that. We had access to their kitchen where we would make juices and in a little garden across the street they had carrots and alfalfa. . . . I had a great cleansing that evening—four tremendous bowel movements—foul smelling. After that I felt like I was on cloud nine.

The roots of toxicity are in the environment, pollutants, the reduction of oxygen in the atmosphere, carcinogens, and in the consequences of modern food production. Toxicity is understood to be a violation of the natural body, a corruption of its internal harmony and balance. In other words, the body is created perfectly, either by nature or God. Without corrupting influences the body's immune system could combat most diseases. Many proponents of cleansing and detoxification therapies such as Jensen argue that pharmaceutical interventions merely suppress the symptoms of this toxicity and may even contribute to it. A college student who had practiced a variety of alternative health regimes told us that she was encountering more people with chronic ailments of various kinds.

> I think this is all new because of the pollutants and contaminants we're absorbing through our skin. Everything is putting such an incredible weight on our bodies. Our bodies are not made to digest and ingest these synthetic chemicals instead of organic ones.

The view that bodies are contaminated and subject to threat is a recurrent theme at CFC meetings, lectures at the local food co-op, meetings of HLQ and Wellness 2000, as well as in our interviews with alternative practitioners and patients. For example, one longtime alternative health activist told a large audience at a CFC meeting that "oxygen depletion leads to cancer." He argued that oxygen depletion is a result of worldwide deforestation and of eating food devoid of enzymes, minerals, and lipids.

The second principle is rejuvenation. This means not the removal of disease but the pursuit of health through nutritional regimes, and mineral and vitamin supplementation, among other modalities. Eating wholesome organic foods in their proper combination is thought to enhance the body's immune system, energy level, and overall sense of well-being. Rejuvenation may also include other alternative modalities such as acupuncture, bodywork, oxidation therapies, and spiritual or meditative approaches.

Rejuvenation, in much of alternative health, refers to the recovery of the aesthetic value of perfect health or well-being. Among all branches of alternative medicine, health refers not only to the absence of disease but also to the achievement of a particular state of being. For example, one specialist in biofeedback and bodywork modalities told us:

> The body has a wonderful wisdom, and it can balance, and you just need to help a little here and there and sit back and watch what's happening, then help a little more when needed.

One speaker at a CFC meeting made the same point but expressed it in more traditionally religious terms:

> There is a healing power within you that is greater than any disease. God made you in his own image. You are not an accident. You are not a random collection of chemicals so that doctors have to come in to cut and poison. God wants you to be on the earth and gave us the ability to heal ourselves. There is something in you greater than any disease you can possibly have.

In these remarks, perfection is understood as not invented or created but recovered. It is not a product of human will and construction but the rediscovery of the inherent nature of things. This recovery is not essentially moral or utilitarian. It does not involve the just regulation of interpersonal conduct or the use of others in the pursuit of self-interest. Unlike a painting or sculpture, this state of being is not a representation of nature but an effort to drive ourselves back to an original condition of balance and harmony.

How is the alternative health regime with its emphasis on "material" interventions connected to more spiritually oriented protocols such as energy medicine, crystal healing, past life regression, and the like? At the extreme end of the continuum spiritual approaches dematerialize illness. Disease is understood purely as an expression of spiritual and psychological states. In other words, a person's psychological condition is such that he is cut off from deeper and wider sources of well-being. But this position is atypical because most practitioners try to weave together in somewhat unstable ways spiritual and "material" protocols. On the one hand detoxification can be expanded to include a process of "spiritual cleansing" of toxic attitudes and values, all of which produce stress that is health destroying. In practice "material" and spiritual cleansing interact with each other providing the condition for the increasing efficacy of the other. On the other hand, rejuvenation in its ideal form amounts to the elimination of the body as a limit, which becomes a transparent medium for high-energy, spiritually enhanced states of being. We call these regimes "aesthetic practices" because their goal is the achievement of a kind of self-perfection, a state of perfect health that is in accord with the perfection of nature. Moreover, the patient works on herself "artfully," with skill and persistence.

Two Cancer Patients and Their Health Regimes

A good example of the path from conventional medicine to an alternative regime and one that reskills the person in the process is the experience of Ann Frahm. Frahm spoke at a CFC meeting recounting her experiences, which were also the subject of her book *The Cancer Battle Plan.*[10] Her experiences are, we believe, paradigmatic of a certain trajectory that reflects the lives of many of the patients we've interviewed. Frahm spoke to three to four hundred people many of whom were cancer patients at the CFC in 1992. After an opening presentation that included a history of the CFC and an attack on the pharmaceutical and medical establishments, Frahm began to tell her story.

Frahm experienced at the age of thirty-four excruciating pain in all her muscles and joints. Her doctor diagnosed the problem as bursitis complicated by a kidney inflection and prescribed "inactivity and antibiotics." But her problems intensified and she wound up taking many medications for pain and to help her sleep. Finally as her condition worsened, she and her husband went to a hospital emergency room. The results of her CaT-scan were reported to her by a young surgeon who said, "I'm late for surgery, Mrs. Frahm. I hate to tell you this but you have advanced breast cancer." In fact her muscle and joint pain was a consequence of tumors that had spread all over her body. She soon underwent a mastectomy as well as chemo and radiation treatment. Then her cancer became resistant to these drugs and she had a bone marrow transplant. Her condition following the transplant was "deemed hopeless."

Frahm describes her path to recovery as a process of removing herself from the control of the medical system and learning about how to rejuvenate her immune system through eating raw fruits and vegetables, continuous juicing, enemas, herbal cleansing and colonics to remove layers of toxicity in the intestinal tract. During this period she sought out a nutritionist well versed in holistic medicine who told her, "First thing you need is to clean out your body." Frahm's problem was located in the liver and colon, which were not working properly because of the buildup of toxicity. Frahm began to address this issue through self-administered enemas—two eight-cup enemas every day. She also experimented with coffee enemas, originally part of the Gerson anti-cancer treatment (Dr. Max Gerson established a famous holistic clinic in Mexico). Because enemas can deplete the "good bacteria" in the intestinal tract she also had to replenish her flora with acidophilus. Frahm also went on a fourteen-day juice fast and felt her energy growing steadily. This required a familiarity with the local health food store where she purchased organic fruits and vegetables. Live foods, which are liquefied through juicing, provide a large amount of enzymes, which are needed for rejuvenation.

A typical day during this period for Frahm involved the following; First, upon waking up, she drank a mixture of two tablespoons of olive oil and four ounces of fresh grapefruit juice. Then she would lie on her right side for twenty minutes with her right knee to her chest to open the pathway to her gall bladder so that the oil and juice could dissolve any stones there. She would also add one teaspoon of fiber cleanse to a glass of juice four times a day as well as drink a glass of distilled water mixed with "green-drink powder" five times a day in order to build blood, oxygenate cells, and destroy free radicals. Other elements of her daily regime included ingesting megadoses of vitamin C powder and drinking an herbal tea. During the day she cooked her meals at low temperatures because heat, as she learned, devitalizes the nutrient value of food. She also learned about the proper combining of food to ensure complete digestion.

Despite the fact that her cancer is now in remission she still follows a less strenuous but still demanding regimen, which she claims is the condition for her continuing good health. She has become a popular speaker and writer on alternative health topics as she deepens her understanding of alternative medicine. During this ordeal what sustained her and gave her the courage to continue even when her condition worsened was her Christian religious faith that God was leading her along the right path.

Frahm has come to understand the cancer is a "disease of civilization" caused by exposure to environmental toxicity, the consumption of high amounts of fat, diary products and meat as well as pesticides, food preservatives, and drugs, and, finally, lifestyles that are high in stress and "unresolved conflict." Consistent with others in the CFC she believes that ultimately disease is a result of violating God's "moral and material law." By this she means that there is a divine plan for healthy living that increasingly modern societies violate. The result is disease.

One other patient who appeared at various times before the CFC had a similar story to tell. Bella was diagnosed with Hodgkin's Lymphoma at eighteen. She went through the usual battery of treatments including chemo and radiation. After another bout of treatment she developed liver cancer and was given two months to live. Desperate, she heard from a friend about the Ernesto Contraros cancer clinic in Mexico. At the clinic she received Laetrile (Amygdalin) treatment as well as retention enemas and B1 shots and has been cancer free for eight years. She told the audience that at the clinic she learned a lot about diet and nutrition and "discovered herself and her self-esteem." She now believes that disease is a result of "external and internal imbalances" including emotions and stress. In order to preserve her health she now eats organic meat, vegetables, and fruits and takes digestive enzymes. She believes in the importance of maintaining acid/alkaline balance but emphasizes the reduction of the acid level.

What stands out in Bella's story is the weight she gives to the beliefs and commitments of the patient as critical in their recovery. "There are many successful cancer cures including chemotherapy. It depends on you and your psychological makeup. My advice is trust your gut and follow your instincts. Make up your mind and do what's right for you and stick with it. Don't try to do everything at once." She believes that the key to her cure was losing her fear, which resulted in "spiritual growth." She ended her story with the mantra of the CFC, "God didn't make any mistakes. We're the ones that screw up." In the context of Bella's entire story, the comment about chemotherapy is somewhat puzzling. But, overall, her point seems to be that one must tailor an alternative health regime to the specific situation and needs of the patient, there must a commitment to following through over a sustained period, a belief that the regime will work and the person will become transformed for the better in the process.

These two examples express common patterns among many of the patients we interviewed. One NLG activist suffered as a child from thyroid enlargement. Her doctor recommended an operation but she experimented with taking kelp or iodine tablets. The improvement in her condition led her to do extensive reading. She developed her own diet that was adapted to her needs and situation. She lost twenty pounds, "and all my energy came back and I've had no problem since." She wonders, though, whether this diet would work with young people because the environment and their personal lives are so different from her own.

Jean suffered from eating disorders, which worsened when she was in her twenties. She came to understand she could address her anorexia disorder through a dietary regime that could provide her with the sense of control over her body she needed but in a way that avoided unhealthy foods with excess sugar that caused her to be depressed and anxious. The diet that she and her holistic nutritionist developed eliminated refined sugars and this eventually led to an interest in macrobiotics. Since we last talked to her she was an active member of a macrobiotic study group where she continued to learn about this Japanese dietary regime and its connection to larger metaphysical belief system. What may be surprising about the application of these regimes to a person's life is that they not only transform the person but also open the person up to the potential for social transformation. Jean was active in the holistic network while the NLG activist considers herself a conservative Christian, and is active in the Christian network. Despite these differences they share a common set of health practices that move them in a similar direction.

Health Practices and the Aesthetic Ideal

What does it mean to talk about the health regime as an aesthetic practice? While we have touched on this subject, we want to explore it here in more depth. We emphasize two constructions of aesthetic creation. The first is the postmodern conception partially expressed in Foucault's work. This project, as some have argued, involves self-creation or self-invention independent of normatively regulated orders.[11] Through the use of creative imagination the person forms herself as a work of art. The goal is the intensification of life in ever greater degrees.

According to Honneth, "[S]uch an aesthetic model of human freedom is what underlies, in one way or another, all versions of a theory of the `postmodern.'" This aesthetic model, Honneth argues, unfolds in two stages, the moment of negative freedom in which the person distances himself from all tradition and community, and the experience of positive freedom or the experimental testing of possible forms of life. This form of experimental self-creation can be found in contemporary music with its hybrid assemblage of diverse musical genres. One example among many is the music of Astor Piazzolla who combines classical music with his native tango to produce a musical form that transgresses conventional boundaries.[12] Edward Said has called this transgressive element the heart of postmodern music.[13] The model of artistic creation as transgressive becomes the model for self-creation. In other words, the self must be constituted through unique combinations of disparate materials available in the culture.

The second construction of aesthetics is an older one that has certain affinities with Plato and with what we call, following others, classical aesthetic theory.[14] This view understands the origins of aesthetic activity in the process of mimesis. Art copies the inherent perfection of nature. There is an inherent order, coherence, and beauty that artists reproduce through imaginative acts. Art is not self-invention but a maeutic process in which the artist serves as the midwife to facilitate the rebirth of the latent order in the world. For example, Michelangelo claimed that he saw in the unmolded clay a preexisting structure that he brought to the surface through his own work. The goal here is not to increase life but to create similarities between the person and the world that can be interpreted as a drive to become identical with the world.

What specifically is the relevance of the classical model of aesthetics to alternative health regimes? To be sure, both aesthetic projects involve a self-mastery of techniques that are learned. But, for the alternative health practitioner, the medium is her own body in a special way that can be understood in terms of classical aesthetic theory. The patient/practitioner works on her body as the artist works on a canvas or other medium in order to rediscover a sense of balance and harmony preexisting in the world. The body becomes a model of a preexisting original. Unlike postmodernist constructions, the prior model is not a copy of a copy that slides toward infinity but an original. The alternative health practitioner's task is to recover the body's latent self-perfection through the midwifery of her regimes.[15]

The classical notion of aesthetics is bound up with the category of the "natural" or its cognate the "organic." The natural, in the discourse of alternative health, means three things. First, what is natural conforms to an original structure of balance and harmony of which the body is a part. In metaphysical branches of alternative health, the body has both nonphysical and physical dimensions that, under optimal conditions, are in harmony. In other alternative health approaches, the body is primarily a physical-biological system that can regulate itself perfectly, unless contaminated by pollution, mineral-deficient food, or other aspects of modern life. Either way, the natural body is a perfect body that exists outside of history and society. Second, the natural is an aesthetic source of guidance and orientation that must be recovered. Because the natural body is outside of history, its perfection (however conceived) can provide a critical standard against which modern eating, dietary, and medical practices can be judged. Third, the natural is not a human creation and operates apart from the process of self-invention. If recovered, it provides safety in a technologically driven world that is understood to be increasingly losing contact with it. The pursuit of the natural, however constructed, can be found throughout new social movements (e.g., ecology, animal rights, and certain versions of radical feminism, that is, identity politics).[16] The natural emerges and remains as a source of orientation for action despite all attempts to eliminate it by defining it as a socially coded text whose terms are continuously reorganized through strategies of deconstruction.[17]

To be sure, postmodern and romantic aesthetic traditions have also worked their way through the understandings and practices of various alternative health approaches. For example, Fuller argues that certain American alternative health traditions are rooted in metaphysical systems that assert the existence of spiritual forces, powers, and realities that are more like agents which enter the individual under certain conditions and transform them. Swedenborgianism, which influenced American metaphysical health traditions such as Christian Science, conceives of a one-way path from spirit to mind to body as the route to health and well-being. The person must become open to the entrance of such forces through hypnotic trances, which derive from the principles of Antoine Mesmer. We find many contemporary versions of this vitalist language of force, energy, and spirit, which breaks away from the view of nature as a text that must be understood and followed.[18] In practice the classical aesthetic and the romantic/postmodern languages are interwoven in the understandings and practices of actors. But in the final analysis the language of balance, harmony, and law-like perfection predominates. This is so because the language of force, energy, and spirit is too indeterminate and arbitrary to give a set direction for alternative health care regimes. Approaches to health that are one-sidedly spiritual tend to have strong affinities with romantic and postmodernist languages. But holistic health approaches, which emphasize mind-body interactions, operate within the classical aesthetic model.

It may seem strange to compare a model of art derived from painting and sculpture to a health regime, but the similarities are striking. First, the classical aesthetic model is grounded in a world view of an intrinsically meaningful world. According to Charles Taylor, the classical view sees the world as a text embodying ideal meanings that orient action.[19] In Taylor's understanding of the classical model, if the text is properly read, it is incorporated into one's life and thus changes it (one's soul becomes aligned with the balances and proportions inherent in the cosmos). In the same way, much of the alternative health literature discusses the necessity of reordering the presently constituted body, damaged by the ravages of progress, with the natural body, which is understood to be intrinsically proportioned. In both cases, a pursuit of a prior order becomes a standard for action. Among the many examples in the alternative health literature is the following from a newsletter that emphasized oxidation approaches and that was decidedly Christian rather than New Age oriented:

> God gave us an immune system that could protect us from cancer, AIDS, tuberculosis and all other disease, but only if it is working correctly. To have it work right, it must have rest, fresh pure air, exercise, good food and proper elimination of toxins. I must also add here that we must NOT put chemicals, poisons, radiation, and antibiotics (or drugs of any kind) in our system.

Another alternative health book, a guide to cleansing, makes the following claim:

> All remedies that have not been taken from Nature, and are not in accordance with her, prove futile; no matter how often, apparently, they may have operated (seemingly) beneficially and effectively. There are too many deceptions here. The injury that inevitably accompanies all unnatural remedies, sooner or later, always comes to the surface and causes them to disappear again, unfortunately after much harm has been done. Such unnatural or not strictly natural remedies come and go, therefore, and never find an abiding place of refuge.

Second, like the pursuit of natural beauty, perfect health is recovered, not invented. Clearly, alternative medicine engages in bodily interventions (e.g., colonics, acupuncture, chelation treatment, and juicing), but these interventions are understood as a peeling away of toxic layers that come from institutional arrangements and practices (e.g., pollution, devitalized foods, drug-based medicine). Once these are stripped away, what remains is a body capable of resisting all disease—a perfect body. One herbalist who also practices naturopathy told us briefly about "layering":

> Holistically speaking, people are layered—things have gone wrong . . . things that have happened to you that have made an impression on your body or mind and then they have been hidden. You've pushed them down so to speak. The "holding it down" always takes energy. So, the healer has to start with what's on top.

In order to get at an underlying condition, the healer must first work through layers of "toxicity" that may come from drugs, improper nutrition, or the stresses of everyday life. Eventually, the underlying condition (that many in alternative medicine believe resides in the colon) is addressed, and the body can return to a state where its self-healing capacities can function. As one practitioner of therapeutic touch put it: "The body heals itself and what we have to do is to set up an environment for healing."

The third correspondence is perhaps the most counterintuitive. How is the pursuit of beauty, inherent in the classical model of aesthetics, applicable to alternative health regimes? How is the external beauty inherent in nature applicable to the creation of a beautiful body? We follow Foucault in his proposal that aesthetics involves not only the creation of beautiful objects but also the creation of a certain kind of person. Most obviously, a healthy person "looks better"—hair, nails, skin, and eyes appear radiant and vibrant. But, more significantly, the classical conception of beauty is one where beauty endures and is not subject to decay. It is therefore connected to the notion of immortality. So too, in alternative health the perfect body appears invulnerable to the point where some claim that the person is potentially immortal:

> The cleansing of the alimentary canal makes it possible to purify the lymphatic system, the blood, the brain and the entire body. You will enjoy greater health, energy, endurance, strength and mental alertness. Expect to live a longer life, looking and feeling good to the end, digesting and assimilating properly the smaller portions of food your body will now require! In fact, you might decide not to die at all and prefer to watch your body become younger instead of older.

A body that is properly balanced and "naturally aligned" is externally beautiful. Beauty in both the classical model and alternative health is the outward expression of a deeper structure of order and balance.

Finally, the recovery of the body's natural order and balance provides a source of safety and security, "a still point in a changing world."[20] Unlike the postmodern aesthetic project where transgression leads to danger and uncertainty, in the classical project the goal is to be grounded in the certainties of nature. In one newsletter, entitled *The Whole Person,* an advocate of "Quantum Process" frames her approach to health, involving deep breathing, as a solution to the uncertainties of modern life:

> Are there simple answers to complex questions? Our lives these days are certainly filled with an assortment of worries, problems and

frustrations. So, much of the quality of living is being compromised, it seems by stress, illness and emotional turmoil which is eroding self esteem and increases the frantic pace of our lives. There's so much information now bombarding us . . . that stress is becoming a constant companion. Wouldn't it be wonderful if there were simple solutions? . . . Right now before you go further, take a deep breath. Thank you! That willingness to take a deep breath is, in fact, where we begin our journey to find those simple answers. (April-May 1992)

"Breath" for this practitioner becomes the symbol of the link between the body and the natural world and a route to the safety of our natural home.

In summary, the alternative health regime, because it is self-administered and uniquely applied, is removed from bureaucratic supervision, in contrast to conventional medicine. Moreover, since the person must "work on him/herself" with knowledge and skill, the process is analogous to Foucault's argument concerning the path of escape from the microphysics of power. It is a technology of the self that is in some sense liberating. In addition, the purpose of this technology is the pursuit of boundless energy, total well-being, balance, and harmony. This is an example of the classical aesthetic project at its core because it aspires to the recovery of a state of bodily perfection that is part of the "wisdom of nature." In summary, the classical aesthetic ideal for alternative health becomes both a source of resistance to the intrusion by institutions and a goal to be reclaimed.

Aesthetics and Politics

Ann Frahm's daily battle with cancer in the form of her self-administered health regime suggests that this search for perfect harmony with nature opens up individuals to wider political involvements. The process of detoxification, enacted daily through various forms of cleansing, taught her that cancer is a "disease of civilization" caused by built-up toxicity and the stresses of daily life. Her quest for an optimal level of health in accordance with God's law led her to become increasingly critical of the obstacles to health that are embedded in the organization of modern societies. What is the connection between the pursuit of harmony with nature through an alternative health regime and the process of becoming open to the need for social transformation?

In order to further analyze this process of politicization we draw upon the work of Nancy Fraser who delineates four meanings attached to the concept of public life. The first, "state related," refers to actions or policies of government and all those links that connect government to groups in society. The second is "accessibility of information," which refers to the extent to which people have access to information allowing them to be public actors. The third meaning refers to discussions about common concerns. In Fraser's words, "It designates a theater in modern societies in which political participation is enacted through talk." Finally, public life may refer to agreements about what is in everyone's mutual interest. In other words, this is the way common concerns are transformed into agreements about how these concerns should be addressed. We will demonstrate how alternative health regimes, which we claim have an aesthetic core, make participants available for public life in the meanings that Fraser identifies.[21]

We want to specify further that the politicizing potential of alternative health care practices has both positive (what some call "liberatory") and negative expressions (called by some "resistance"). By "negative" we mean external obstacles that block the purposes and intentions of actors. By "positive" we mean the pursuit and achievement of generalizable goals that can be shared. We note here that we are using the terms *positive* and *negative* from the viewpoint of alternative health participants rather than observers. While alternative health in the abstract engages each of these four meanings of public life both positively and negatively, our interest is in the way participants understand and relate to these various dimensions of public life. In other words, the connection of alternative health to public life can be comprehended in two ways: as an obstacle to the achievement of goals (negative expression) and as goals and purposes that can be shared and pursued (positive expression). Alternative health participants interact with public life in ambivalent and contradictory ways, but it is possible to identify central directions with respect to their public orientations.

Alternative health care practices are bound up with the policies of the state, largely in a negative sense—the state as an obstacle, a variant of Habermas's "colonization of the lifeworld." Through regulation and at times suppression of health care practitioners and health products (including technology), the state is seen as an obstacle to the practice of alternative health regimes. In addition, with respect to the second category—information and its dissemination—the state is understood in a negative sense as limiting and at times suppressing the availability of information about alternative health. It is important to note that some in alternative health recognize the need for a degree of regulation and licensing of alternative health practitioners, but this position is not the dominant one in the alternative health community.

One chiropractor who is active in the alternative health community complained to us,

> The political environment [for alternative medicine] is terrible. I mean this new thing with the FDA that's coming in . . . you know, basically to take peoples's right to take care of themselves away from them, I mean, they can't buy a vitamin in a dose that's higher than the RDA, and the RDA is laughable. . . . Between the IRS and the FDA, I feel like I'm living in a Kafka novel.

This practitioner is referring to the effort a few years ago by the Federal Food and Drug Administration (FDA) to redefine certain vitamins and other natural food substances as drugs and therefore only available through doctors' prescriptions. In addition, this sense of government suppression was intensified by a 1992 incident in which the clinic of a prominent holistic M.D. was raided by armed FDA agents who confiscated a supply of natural substances as well as files and temporarily closed the clinic. Many of the people we interviewed mentioned this incident, and it was discussed at CFC meetings as well as National Health Federation conventions.

CFC meetings, after the opening prayer, are followed by brief presentations outlining legislative initiatives of concern to the alternative health community. One such concern discussed at a recent meeting was a proposed bill in the Pennsylvania legislature that would recognize only registered dieticians as nutritional counselors. Speakers also urged participants to support legislation that would allow terminally ill patients to "receive the same treatments in the United States that people are receiving in Mexico and Canada."

A common theme at the CFC lectures and the food co-op is the suppression of information about alternative health modalities. For example, one advocate of oxidation therapies asserted that pharmaceutical companies and the government have directly suppressed information about the benefits of "ozone therapy." He claimed that the FDA and pharmaceutical companies have access to scientific papers showing the value of this therapy but refuse to accept it and make it public.

We extend Fraser's notion of "state related" to include health care institutions with close connections to the state: pharmaceutical companies, hospitals, and the medical profession (licensed and regulated by the state). Alternative health participants come to understand that the roots of illness are in these basic health care institutions of modern societies. In other words, biomedicine is thought to be imposed upon people without allowing a choice of alternatives. One CFC activist put it this way:

> You know they say we have freedom in this country. We don't have freedom. How much freedom do I have to see the kind of doctor that I want? And how much freedom does that doctor have to practice here? None! And then they say we have freedom! And I don't think there's any freedom more important than that freedom—taking care of yourself the way you want to.

Detoxification means, in part, the removal of the effects of conventional medicine—primarily drugs. Drugs are seen as foreign substances that violate the body's natural harmony. One practitioner discussed the harmful effects of prescription drugs with respect to diabetes,

> They're [doctors] managing the symptoms. And the doctor's gonna manage the symptoms by saying, "Well, let's give you the medication either by mouth or by injection depending on what your blood sugars are by monitoring your blood sugar at home through blood and let's give you the drug to stop the sugar process." Well, okay . . . I'm taking this foreign substance into my mouth, I am going to digest this, it is then going to go and do something to my pancreas, and then if it's too strong it's still in my system. . . . What happens if it's not digested down properly? Where does the rest of it go? How does it get metabolized and down into the liver . . . and what does it do to those liver cells? Does it cause cancer and does it cause heart disease?

In this conflict with the state and related institutions, the aesthetic understanding of the body becomes the source of resistance to a process of "colonization" by state and economic institutions.

How is this aesthetic conception of the body and its grounding in the natural a source of resistance to "colonization" in Habermas's sense? Activists resist and criticize the effects of "progress" through an experience with alternative health regimes that is in turn grounded in a view of the natural body. In this resistance we see a play of oppositions: the natural versus the artificial, the pure versus the contaminated, the original versus the constructed, hubris versus humility (or stewardship). Much of this opposition to progress coalesces around opposition to drugs. Drugs are considered an artificially created rather than natural substance, something that contaminates the purity of the body, and an expression of the hubris of biomedicine in its claim to suspend natural principles. One chiropractor told us:

> The patients I see are fed up with doctors—too much specialization, too many drugs. I tell them, "If you quit taking half your medications, you'll feel better." Their livers and kidneys are overloaded.

Another practitioner emphasized the side effects of drugs and, implicitly, the hubris of interventionist medicine.

> Most doctors are honest. They try to give you the right medication. The problem is with pharmaceuticals themselves. They are so side-effect laden, and the patient takes medication and a side effect develops. Then they need a medication for the side effect; that which is given for the side effects develops a side effect and you have a chain reaction.

One patient engaged in a macrobiotic regime told us that she valued the natural herbs she remembered from childhood over the medications prescribed for her by her doctor.

> I mean a cooking class to me is more valuable than taking a bottle of pills if you can cook to heal yourself. I remember what my mother told me about how my grandmother used to pull herbs from her garden to make spring tonic, and they were never sick.

This woman, with a serious chronic illness, told us, "I replaced an addiction to drugs with an addiction to exercise—jogging, aerobics, the rest. Now I have more balance. It all comes down to balance."

The last two aspects of public life are in large part positive because they involve sharing information about what people have to do (the technologies they must learn and practice) and disseminating models of what they can become (perfect health). In both senses, the practice of alternative health constitutes a public. The word "public" should not be construed to mean only a broad homogeneous community in which people address common concerns and form a consensus about common purposes. Fraser has argued that this dominant conception of the "public sphere" occludes the existence of "subaltern publics."[22] A subaltern public is a space that allows for the development of discourses that oppose dominant institutions. In other words, the public is constituted not by one but by many voices. This does not mean that subaltern publics, including alternative health, are permanently balkanized. Subaltern publics are "public" because they are oriented beyond their own context and have the potential to contribute to a societal-wide consensus about the merit and purpose of their values and practices. In this sense, alternative health communities can be construed as a subaltern public with its own distinctive voice and yet raise issues that have more generalizable potential.

The aesthetic ideal of total well-being has politicizing as well as depoliticizing potential with respect to the constitution and enlargement of public spaces. On the one hand, some argue that the full achievement of perfect health is impossible without the reorganization of dominant institutions. On the other hand, some believe that through their own autonomous practices individuals can achieve their goal without changing dominant institutions. In this way, what they pursue leads them away from public life. We can conceptualize these two stances as two poles in a spectrum of possibilities.

Many of the practitioners in the holistic health network we interviewed told us that the key to health is a change in lifestyle and attitude. One herbalist said, "Nothing happens to you. You're doing something wrong and we have to figure out what you're doing wrong." Another practitioner told us that patients "heal themselves" by becoming aware of habits, thought patterns, and attitudes that are self-destructive. Others recognized that institutional arrangements must be challenged but asserted that "politicians and politics are corrupt" and that "I don't have the energy to be involved in politics."

At the other end of the spectrum, some activists seemed to project the model of the natural body in imagining an ideal society. At one Wellness 2000 meeting attended by ecology activists, alternative health practitioners, and others, the topic of personal health soon expanded to include discussions of "sustainable systems," "bioregions," and "living off the land." Participants asserted that "progress has made things worse" and we have "an information overload." One participant observed that throughout the country people are engaged in "spontaneous projects," such as organic gardening and "ecologically sound agriculture," in order to recover a radically new relationship with the world. This same individual said, "People are trying to reinvigorate the sensual qualities of the world—the beauty of the world." The model embedded in this discussion is one of recovering harmonious rather than instrumental interactions with the natural world. Just as the ancient Greeks thought that there was a relationship between beauty in a person's life and beauty in the "polis," so too some health activists see a connection between a conception of personal "beauty" (in accordance with natural principles) and a conception of societal and ecological "beauty" (harmony or balance).

The potential for context-transcending expansion beyond alternative health groups is anticipated and even struggled for by many we interviewed. As the reader may recall, Art Sutton, founder of HLQ, is trying to bring together "social justice movements," ecology groups, and holistic health groups in a coalition called "Wellness 2000." One flyer put out by HLQ lists the following missions as part of this umbrella organization: "holistic health, life skills and lifestyle simplicity, citizen activism, earth stewardship, faith and spiritual disciplines and service to others." Recently, HLQ sponsored an event that recognized the contributions of activists in each of these categories. HLQ has also been instrumental in forging an alliance with the Greens, an ecologically oriented party seeking to bring issues of sustainable economic development to the wider public. For the most part, the idea of a Green party evoked favorable responses from the people we interviewed. Here we see a subaltern public creating links with other subaltern publics and to society as a whole.

In summary, aesthetic constructions of the body provide a critical standard that enables participants to resist the imposition of institutional arrangements on the alternative health community (colonization) and an ideal of an alternative world, grounded in the aesthetic principles of harmony and balance. This ideal is the basis of a critique of progress based on instrumental relations to nature and economic growth.

The experience of alternative health regimes places people in a situation where not being politically involved leaves unresolved the contradiction between their own bodily health practices and the world. People experience constraints (pollution, devitalized food, pesticides) that make it more difficult to pursue their goals of health. The daily experience of these constraints reminds people that something in society is not right—by not becoming involved they are living in a contradictory state. In other words, they are available for movements. They are open to arguments that institutions need to change, but they may not, for various reasons, act on these understandings. This availability does not go away, because it is rooted in their own illnesses and incomplete efforts to get well. In this sense, availability for movements is permanent and may not be fleeting like other concerns.

The Weak Public Sphere

The openness to politicization that technologies of the self promote can be more fully comprehended by drawing upon Nancy Fraser's distinction between a weak and a strong public sphere. For Fraser a weak public sphere consists of unstructured flows of communication, information, and, we would add, images through which interpretations of the world are formed, new needs are generated, and collective identities emerge. Fraser contrasts this with a strong public sphere in which arguments and opinions are directly bound to processes of decision making. A model for the strong public sphere is a parliamentary body.[23] The images of reconciliation with nature that technologies of the self embody circulate within the weak public sphere in the form of images and suggestions, which encapsulate utopian energies. Through the evocation of the natural in dress, conversation, the use of herbs and organic food, flashes of reconciliation with the world are suggested. These flashes of reconciliation surround the arguments, opinions, observations, jokes, and stories that circulate wildly in subaltern alternative health networks.

The alternative health movement's significance may be in its reconstruction of the meaning of illness beyond a narrow medical category. Instead, illness becomes both a representation of the increasing risks of modern societies and the source of bodily and self-transformation that points to other possible worlds. The body both means something and allows us to do something. In other words, the diseased body in alternative health registers a "revenge of nature" in the form of increasing environmental threats and institutional damage. These threats are addressed by technologies of the self that pursue an original body. This original body, aesthetic in its core meaning, points to a new relationship between the person and the world.

Our reconceptualization of alternative health and the weak public sphere allows us to point to a deeper process of politicization than we have previously argued. Whether alternative health regimes lead people to focus on self or social transformation is at this level not relevant, for even personal involvement retains images of reconciliation that can be taken up by movements within the strong public sphere. The concept of weak public sphere connects bodily practices and the notion of the aura to social movements and decision making within the institutional spheres of society. Without the energy at the base of the system, alternative health would lose its character as a popular movement with a weak messianic promise. It would be absorbed into the polity as another interest group or absorbed by biomedicine as a "complementary" addition to its central protocols. In the next chapter we will flesh out this relay between the weak and strong publics and show how they mutually condition and transform one another.

CHAPTER 5

New Social Movements

In this chapter we discuss how social movements draw upon the images and practices that circulate in "the weak public sphere" as the basis for cultural innovation and, more actively, as sites of resistance to dominant institutions. In this light we examine alternative health as a "new social movement"(NSM).[1] We explore the creation of oppositional identities and meanings and argue that the larger significance of alternative health is as a site in which diverse communities and discourses transform one another and challenge a leading expression of what Jürgen Habermas has called the "colonization of the lifeworld." We suggest that in the domain of health there is a partial recognition of precisely the phenomenon to which Habermas's theory refers: the reduction of people to objects in a health care system that regulates them without their understanding or active participation. Advanced technology, interventionist medical procedures, and profit-oriented, bureaucratically administered institutions, as we have noted earlier, dominate this system. The often explicit demand within the alternative health community that health care should be, at least in part, dedifferentiated—returned to a more organic relationship with vernacular healing traditions and with communities—is often coupled with a critique of a system that largely ignores the meaning of health and illness, treating illness as a phenomenon disconnected from the rest of the person. To reconnect health and illness to the lifeworld is, we argue, a chief demand of both wings of the alternative health movement we have studied.

We draw on the work of Habermas who has argued that the source of new social movements is the resistance to the "colonization of the lifeworld" by the media of money and power. Habermas argues that modernity has differentiated three value spheres that had been undifferentiated in premodern societies: the cognitive-instrumental sphere, morality and ethics, and art and aesthetics. But the "developmental logic" of modern societies has created an imbalance. This imbalance was produced by the rise of capitalism and its work ethic with its emphasis on instrumental rationality. The notion of "the system" can be understood in this context. It refers to the way human interactions are governed not by the communicative efforts of participants but by impersonal media of wealth and power. The word *media* means that human interactions are coordinated behind the backs of participants. The market, for example, coordinates interactions free of norms and conscious human planning and produces consequences that can only be identified post hoc by observers. In this sense media delinguistify human interaction. Power can be understood in an analogous form as something that in the last instance coordinates people through the process of bureaucratization. The logic of the system then becomes how the media of power and money operate through the domains of the state and the economy and become more complex and dense in their interactions. Such a developmental logic allows greater mastery of technical tasks in the service of the material reproduction of society and therefore a greater system rationalization.

However, unlike Weber, Habermas does not reduce rationality to its functional and instrumental dimensions. Habermas has a more comprehensive view of rationality which locates it in the lifeworld and communicative efforts of people to come to an agreement through discussion and if need be argumentation. Rationalization at this level refers to the extent to which norms, values, and purposes are not predecided by traditions but are taken up by actors themselves who raise and argue over cognitive, moral, and aesthetic validity claims. The lifeworld becomes more rational, in this sense, insofar as it is more freely coordinated without force. That is, it involves communication without domination.

Colonization, for Habermas, refers to how these two levels of society and their distinct modes of rationalization interact. Colonization refers to the disruption of the ability of people to come to an understanding of their world and to actively coordinate their behavior in light of it. Instead, the media of power and money replace communicative rationality with impersonal coordination that steers people behind their backs. Through this occupation by "the system" social life becomes reified, assuming a thing-like form that withdraws it from human understanding and conscious purpose.[2]

What is the motor propelling colonization? Habermas relies on the writings of Marx to understand the forces behind colonization. For Habermas, as with Marx, capitalism produces economic crises ultimately rooted in the class system. These crises are both managed and displaced by the state through Keynesian crisis-avoiding strategies, which serve to diffuse class conflict. What occurs here is that the state attempts to redistribute wealth to reduce the inequalities created by the class system, which lead to economic problems such as overproduction. As the state extends its management of the economy, economic crises become displaced into the political system. Various people along with Habermas have characterized this displacement as a "rationality crisis." One formulation is that the state is compelled to manage the economy but cannot do so successfully because the resources it needs to do this are blocked by the economic system itself. For example, the state must, on the one hand, provide the conditions for the accumulation of capital and at the same time manage the social consequences that result from accumulation in the form of unemployment, pollution, the retraining of the workforce among other things. But the state cannot extract sufficient resources to meet both functions simultaneously. This vise that the state is in becomes the source of a motivational crisis. People perceive that the government doesn't work well even as they fail to understand the class basis for this political malfunctioning. This leads to what Habermas calls the crisis of state legitimacy.[3]

What interests us here in this thesis is how the expansion of state activity that is both called for and blocked by the capitalist system, leads to the bureaucratization and commodification of the lifeworld. The state encourages the accumulation of capital, which leads to the increasing commodification of everyday life and must manage the effects of that commodification and therefore increases the bureaucratization of everyday life. As a result, people are increasingly reduced to the status of clients and consumers. We can illustrate this by looking at the health care system. As bureaucracies shape medical practices, they make them more technical and unavailable to the practical knowledge of actors. Dying, for example, becomes a statistical and medical event, defined and managed by experts and state agencies, rather than a culturally enacted event. At the same time the health care system becomes more commodified as the result of pressures to use more sophisticated technology with high economic payoffs and through the extension of the corporate model to health care.

In addition, Habermas refers to the realm of family law as an interesting illustration of colonization. Here, although there are progressive elements including the reduction of domestic violence, overall family relations become reified as they are increasingly organized into a legal setting. Instead of addressing family problems themselves, actors become objects in a world governed by experts and often in accordance with laws not understood by participants themselves.[4] This process of colonization encourages family members to act strategically toward one another and therefore break bonds of solidarity.

For Habermas, new social movements can be understood as emerging in the "seams" between lifeworld and system. In other words, new social movements arise in the context of the deepening of commodification and bureaucratization, which are the two forms in which colonization interrupts the symbolic reproduction of the lifeworld. Social movements such as feminism, ecology, gay rights, and civil rights take up new themes such as autonomy, alternative lifestyles, human rights, identity, democratic participation, and self-realization which can be understood as distinct from the direct distribution of wealth and power that were at the heart of the "old" social movements related to class conflict. Habermas conceptualizes new social movements in terms of whether they are offensive or defensive in character. Offensive new social movements seek to extend the processes of rationalization within the lifeworld through the creation of new forms of life, such as efforts to create new family structures, and ecologically sustainable communities and lifestyles. Defensive new social movements seek to defend traditional ways of life, real or imagined, or to defend "new ways of cooperating and living together."[5] Ethnic movements that seek to restore ancient claims, traditions, and practices to an "authentic past" is one example of a defensive stance while intentional communities that try to reinvent the notions of community and family are an example of a more offensive resistance to colonization. Intentional communities resist the bureaucratic supervision of family and community life by insisting on their own autonomy and independent self-management.

Habermas's account of colonization falls short of explaining the face-to-face interactions that lead to new oppositional identities and meanings, in other words, the sociological genesis of new social movements. Alberto Melucci is helpful in this respect. Melucci has focused on the process of meaning and identity formation in social movements. His point of departure is a critique of a reified notion of social movements that views them as a "unified empirical datum."[6] Instead of seeing movements as rational actors or as consequences of structural changes, Melucci views them as processes, lying largely beneath the level of visible political events. These submerged networks, common among peace, feminist, ecology, and other new social movements cannot be understood on a strategic level—as goal-oriented, preference-maximizing actors. Instead, for these new social movements, an organization is not simply a means for attaining goals but is an arena in which "actors self-consciously practice in the present the future changes they seek." They function as "cultural laboratories" in which participants experiment with new cultural codes and ways of life. Rather than emphasizing structural change, these submerged networks are more interested in everyday life and its autonomy.

In this chapter we combine both elements of new social movement theory—Habermas's colonization theory and Melucci's focus on the emergence of new meanings and "collective identities" in submerged networks.[7] We explore the two submerged networks discussed previously and argue that alternative health consists not only of submerged networks similar to others in the peace and feminist movement, for example, but also that it differs in important ways from other new social movement networks.[8] After all, illness (especially chronic illness) is largely resistant to the changing social and political circumstances that shape other forms of discontent. Eating, and its associated rituals, is an activity that is a permanent if not central aspect of everyday life. These differences are significant, for alternative health has important implications for other new social movements and is an important cultural resource for them.

Alternative Health as a Social Movement

A central question is whether we can usefully understand this phenomenon as a social movement. Is alternative health a niche in the health market, a professional movement whose aim is to reform medical and other health professions or to make room for new health professions, a component of other social movements such as the cultural communities loosely known as New Age or the feminist health movement?

According to Melucci, a social movement involves internal soli- darity, conflict with an adversary, and "breaking the limits of compati- bility of the system," which suggests the presentation of demands that would require fundamental structural changes.[9] Submerged networks are "cultural laboratories," largely invisible since they are embedded in everyday life and not openly engaged in political acts such as demon- strations, sit-ins, petitioning, and the like. They are fragmented in the sense that diverse groups with common goals often have only tenuous relationships with one another and that submerged networks are tem- porary in duration. Individuals move in and out of these networks, rather than being totally committed to them. Submerged networks may or may not break out into the political sphere, into open contestation with authorities. They are therefore an important resource for social movements but cannot themselves be considered a social movement.[10]

We would suggest that alternative health operates simultaneously on two levels—as a social movement with an organized interest group dimension and in submerged social movement networks. Claus Offe has distinguished three levels of power in modern societies: the level of political elites, a second level in which interest groups and other collectivities form coalitions with or oppose one another in contesting for resources and in defining the terms of political debate, and, finally, a third arena that can best be understood as rooted in everyday inter- actions.[11] As Habermas explains it:

> In the lower arena conflicts are not directly for money or power but rather for definitions. At issue are the integrity and autonomy of lifestyles, perhaps the protection of traditionally established subcul- tures or changes in the grammar of traditional forms of life. Regionalist movements are examples of the former, feminist or eco- logical movements examples of the latter. For the most part these battles remain latent; they take place within the microsphere of everyday communication, and only now and then do they consolidate into public discourses and higher-level forms of intersubjectivity.[12]

Much of the activity of alternative health is on this everyday level. Participants seek to create and sustain a form of life that lies outside of conventional cultural codes and institutional arrangements: in organic farming, cooperative stores, study groups, health fairs, cooking classes, and lectures in which unconventional health information is shared. These and related activities do not involve a high degree of solidarity in order to challenge elites or authorities, but they are a significant

source of new meanings and identities that may have important implications in the more conventionally political arena.

David Eisenberg and others have demonstrated that alternative
health is more than a movement among health professionals: it is a
popular phenomenon. More than forty billion dollars is spent per year
by health consumers for alternative health treatment (most of which is
out of pocket). Moreover, in this third level, as we have shown, practitioners, patients, and activists coexist in a community where the gap
in prestige and knowledge between expert and client is rather narrow.
Rather than being a phenomenon of the New Age, what is most significant about alternative health is that it includes diverse communities
and discourses.

While much of alternative health exists within this "third arena," it
breaks through into the second level as well. There are lobbying
groups that represent particular alternative health interests from naturopathy to macrobiotics (for example, the Kushi Institute), whose
interest is to challenge legislative efforts to restrict their freedom of
action. There are professional associations such as the Nurse Healers
Professional Associates, largely sympathetic to alternative health
(helping to publicize therapeutic touch among other alternative modalities). The American Holistic Medical Association (AHMA) is one such
professional association for the small number of committed holistic
physicians. In addition to these groups, the National Health Federation
is a lobbying and promotional organization for alternative health on
the national level. It also publishes a national newsletter and holds
yearly "health expos" where alternative practitioners can promote
themselves and share information with others. These groups operate in
the second arena in which there are explicit efforts to contest for
resources, form coalitions, influence legislation, reform particular professions, fight for the existence of new ones, educate the public, and
the like.

Two Alternative Health Networks Revisited

Alternative health is a site in which diverse groups find a common
basis for renewal and sustain a critique of the system. Given Melucci's
caution not to reify social movements but to account for their diverse
and often contradictory components, we examine the diversity of the
alternative health terrain in Pittsburgh. In contrast to those who see a
"cultural war" in America between cultural progressives and the

Christian right we have discovered a site where the two meet and share common concerns and resistances.[13]

The holistic health network, as discussed earlier, centers around a Pittsburgh-based set of groups. Of the many local practitioners, occasional health fairs, meetings, workshops, lectures, retreats, and study groups, we have located three sites or network "nodes" that draw a clientele or constituency from throughout the Pittsburgh area and that are widely known in the alternative health community.

First, there is the food co-op, which is the only one in the city. In addition to its selection of organic fruits and vegetables, the co-op also contains a small café where many of the "regulars" hang out. It functions as a "third place"—a region between home and work that provides an alternative to the impersonality of the workplace and supermarkets as well as the privacy and (for some) the loneliness of the private sphere.[14] The co-op also sponsors a weekly lecture series on alternative health, which draws between fifteen and thirty people. Topics range from homeopathy, naturopathy, herbal treatments, vegetarian cooking classes, "Making Mineral Preparations," "Reflexology," "Alexander Technique," "Psychology of Wellness," "Responsible Investing," and "Nontoxic Zoning and Remodeling." According to one of the full-time staff members, who has been employed there longer than any other employee, co-op shoppers have, over the past few years, become a more diverse group with more elderly and African Americans making regular appearances in addition to the "hippie types." She observed, "Many super mainstream people are coming here. They're not alternative-looking people." While expressing a good deal of satisfaction in her work, this staff member observed,

> It's psychologically hard to work here because most of the people who come through here are looking for different answers and [they are] people who are not well. They have some kind of problem and they're trying to work it out in their lives.

This same staff member described the typical shopper as suffering from physical problems as well as "feelings of isolation." Perhaps using her own experiences as a model (she started at the co-op while suffering from chronic fatigue syndrome and desperately searching for a cure), she described the co-op regulars as "a little odd—like touched. It's not that people understand you but you can talk about what your views are and how you feel." This is not, in other words, your typical grocery store.

The second node is Holistic Living Quest (HLQ), a group that distributes a monthly mailing and newsletter about alternative health and, more broadly, personal growth, wellness, and progressive political activities. Thus, HLQ is a clearinghouse for information about alternative health activities in Pittsburgh and the surrounding area. Art Sutton, the founder of HLQ, with the help of a board of directors and volunteers, puts out a directory of alternative health services (the directory has now expanded to include citizen activist groups, family and gender issues, progressive religious and spiritual disciplines, and ecology groups, among other topics), as well as its monthly newsletter and mailing. The mailing (to more than three thousand people) includes flyers and advertisements from a wide range of health practitioners, activist groups, and religious and spiritual organizations that pay HLQ a small fee for access to the mailing list. As discussed earlier, Art Sutton sees his mission as facilitating the work of others whom he sees as part of a "holistic living community."

In 1996, HLQ sponsored a series of meetings in which alternative health activists and others were invited to respond to a series of proposals by the HLQ board of directors ("Wellness 2000"). Participating in these meetings were alternative health practitioners, a witch and goddess worshiper, a Green Party activist, a director of an institute specializing in bodywork modalities, advocates of Christian mysticism (from the Edgar Cayce Institute), a progressive Catholic priest, a holistically oriented nurse, an ecology activist interested in "sustainable systems," a professional therapist, and an astrologer, to name only a few. Among other things, the Wellness 2000 proposal calls for closer links to feminist, ecology, and citizen activist groups, fundraising for a "movement center" where participants can "socialize and exchange ideas," development of a regional education and healing center, a regional barter-for-service program, a certificate program to "facilitate individuals' venturing into wellness-oriented careers," and development of a health maintenance organization involving natural and alternative practitioners.

Over the six years of Wellness 2000's existence they achieved some of their goals but not others. Part of the difficulty was that the goals themselves were both ambitious and contradictory. On the one hand, the effort to develop a health maintenance organization for alternative practitioners required a degree of official recognition and funding that was not available, at least not in Pittsburgh. Art's idea was that the HMO would be modeled after the European health spa. Patients would pay a yearly membership fee and get a specified amount of alternative health service from the wide range of practitioners working in the HMO. Despite considerable effort, Art gave up both on this idea and the development of a "regional movement center."

Art's vision for Wellness 2000 was for this organization to (1) advance alternative health's official recognition and professionalization; (2) establish closer links between various therapies and in doing so solidify a collective identity (Art regarded alternative health's identity as rather weak, in part because of the strong individualist orientation of practitioners and patients); and (3) establish links between alternative health and other movements for change including religiously based social justice movements, ecology, labor groups, among others. But the problem was that very few of the participants of Wellness 2000 shared the entire vision. Most were not interested in establishing links with other social movements on the formal level (rather than the informal networking we will soon discuss). One practitioner we talked to worried that these efforts might erode the strength of alternative health; its diversity and close association with patients' everyday concerns. In addition, Art's partial sympathy with the political projects of social justice movements was not widely shared.

Wellness 2000 did achieve some success in creating a "speaker's bureau" and its idea of developing a new profession of "wellness educator," a paraprofessional who would mediate between patients, doctors, and alternative practitioners, has received some interest. But, the ambitious goal (the alternative HMO) of achieving greater institutional recognition not primarily through integration with biomedicine but through the establishment of a kind of parallel system where alternative medicine would compete with biomedicine was bound to be a difficult one to achieve. In addition, the goal of creating formal links with other social movements in order to more closely associate alternative health with progressive social justice movements, lacked internal support and, in some respects, ran counter to the first goal of achieving greater official recognition.

Six years after Wellness 2000 was created, Art gave up on the project. He told us, somewhat dejectedly, that it required too much energy, implying that he did not receive enough help from others, and that much of what he tried to accomplish would happen anyway, given the successes of alternative health. Art's overall goal of "seeding or pushing the process," of educating people about "holistic living" was already happening and no longer required an organization such as Wellness 2000. He has also learned to modify his own vision so that it is in more accord with "what is possible."

I've learned to have visions but not turn them into goals. I want to be much more patient. . . . I have the same vision today as five years ago but back then I would have been trying to make it happen and now I'm learning what can happen now and what can't happen now. I'm starting to work better with what's presented to me now rather than what I want to create now. It caused a lot of frustration, a lot of frustration.

The third node in the holistic network is an eclectic, alternative health–oriented practice located in the heart of Pittsburgh. The energetic and entrepreneurial director, trained in macrobiotics and "attitudinal healing," provides macrobiotic and nutritional counseling to a clientele that has been steadily increasing since the practice began in 1985. In addition to individual counseling there are also workshops, classes, a study group, and self-help groups available on a range of topics: "spiritual dimensions of weight loss," shiatsu massage, "yogatherapy," Chinese astrology, a class in "natural immunity," macrobiotics, and a "Kids' Workshop for Self-Esteem." The director, guest instructors, or one of the two full-time staff members runs classes and workshops.

The director of this alternative health practice estimates that 80 percent of her clients are women, primarily middle class and well educated, although this gender and class composition is a fairly recent development. She estimates that the vast majority of her patients come to her because of a serious illness, often terminal. But she has made a conscious effort to "attract more mainstream clientele" with classes, workshops, and self-help groups. Over the past few years since we first interviewed the director of this practice and observed some of her programs, she has achieved considerable success in attracting a more mainstream clientele. She has expanded her staff, the range of programs offered, and her physical facilities now include a number of floors in an office building.

The second major network is located in a working-class suburb north of Pittsburgh. Members are largely (although by no means entirely) "conservative Christians" (the term used by one of the leaders of the group). A cancer survivor and her husband, a sanitary engineer, founded the CFC twenty years ago. The name comes from a movement that began in 1975 to support a doctor who was put on trial for offering alternative cancer treatments in California. Throughout the country, support groups for this doctor formed and the one in the Pittsburgh area affiliated with this movement. Now the only one of the original groups left is the one in the Pittsburgh area. While rooted in the local community and informally tied to the local Methodist Church, it does not have any official affiliation with a church.

The people who provide most of the day-to-day leadership of the group are a married couple, a retired steel worker and his wife (Ed and Sandra), a woman who has been active in the NHF for many years—and the husband of the woman who had breast cancer and whose search for alternative treatment led to the creation of this group. The formal "director" of the group is a chiropractor whose practice has little to do with traditional chiropractic techniques and instead utilizes a range of alternative modalities to treat patients with various chronic ailments.

Since its inception, the CFC has held monthly meetings that are attended by 120–400 people. Meetings open with a prayer and feature a speaker, often brought in from outside the city, who explains some alternative approach to treating chronic disease. Patient testimonials are also quite common. In one instance, a cancer survivor, who has written a book on her experience, recounted to more than four hundred people her ordeal and eventual cure through alternative treatments. Recently, to celebrate the twentieth anniversary of the group, a prominent holistic physician gave a lecture at a CFC meeting attended by more than 350 people. Typically, one hour is devoted to questions from the audience. In many cases, questioners are suffering from a chronic disease and use this opportunity to tell the audience of their experiences, often involving unhappy and at times tragic encounters with the medical system. It is common for participants at the meeting to exchange phone numbers and to make themselves available to others in order to spread information about their own experiences and share their knowledge. Often whole families will attend, and it not uncommon to see two or three generations of a family sitting together listening to a speaker and often taking notes or tape recording the lecture. The sharing of these "sad stories" about conventional medicine helps to build the rudiments of a collective identity.

While the founders of this group are committed Christians for whom Christianity is a world view and a guide to living, this is not a group devoted to faith healing or to the other spiritually oriented healing approaches associated with various Protestant sects (such as Pentecostalism and Christian Science). Instead, the dominant alternative health philosophy espoused by the leadership of the group is naturopathy, emphasizing nutritional treatment for disease and a nutritional regime for preventing disease. Moreover, the colon is understood as the origin for most disease, and most speakers recommend frequent colon cleansing.

Of the seventy-four people surveyed at a recent CFC meeting (114 attended the meeting), the average age is fifty-nine, and only 20 percent are college graduates (approximately half of the seventy-four people attending were members of the CFC). Most characterize themselves as Christians and go to church at least once a week. More than one-third are retired or are full-time housewives. Of those who are employed outside the home, the vast majority are clerical or blue-collar workers. The average household income of CFC members surveyed is $24,800, below the national average and substantially lower than the consumers of alternative medicine sampled in Eisenberg's study.

The central node or site in this network is the monthly meeting but there are also activities that draw subgroups from the CFC. One of these nodes is the local NHF chapter, whose leader is on the NHF national board of directors and is closely affiliated with the CFC. Another node consists of an alternative health group that also meets monthly in the same northern suburb, the NLG. This group sponsors lectures, which emphasize nutrition as well as alternative medicine. Many members of this group, which has been meeting regularly since 1955, also attend CFC meetings.

The NLG has been in continuous operation since 1955 when it was part of a national organization centered in Texas (Natural Foods Associates). The Pittsburgh area NLG got started when its founder, worried about the difficulties she was having with her pregnancies, experimented with organic diary products grown on her friend's farm. At the same time, an osteopath, finding that his patients had a hard time sticking to the dietary regime he recommended, came up with the idea of a patient support group. The two of them joined together with a National Health Federation activist to start the Natural Foods Group (they later changed their name). This was well before the alternative food movement in the late 1960s, so fresh organic food was not readily available. As a result, one of the first activities of the new group was to form their own organic food co-op. They would have a yearly festival at a local community college, which attracted hundreds of people from all over the area. Years later, the co-op is no longer needed but they continue to meet once a month and have branched out to address topics beyond nutrition.

Comparing the Two Networks

What is the relationship between these two networks? What do these networks have in common and how do they differ? The core members of the holistic health network (co-op staff members and volunteers, participants in the macrobiotic study group, activists and practitioners in the HLQ circle, and alternative health practitioners) are primarily white, college educated, and female. But there is a much larger base consisting of occasional co-op shoppers, clients who attend some self-help groups (classes on shiatsu, for example), participants at occasional workshops and lectures, and patients of a variety of alternative practitioners. Most people attending CFC meetings are from blue-collar working-class backgrounds or are self-employed and are considerably older than the participants in the holistic health network.

The social and cultural differences between these two networks are apparent. There is little overlap between CFC members and those on the HLQ mailing list (according to both Art, the HLQ director, and Ed, one of the CFC leaders) and few members of the holistic health network attend CFC meetings. When asked whether she would like to attend any CFC meetings, one nurse, who practices therapeutic touch and has undergone shamanic training, replied, "I'm not sure. Some of them think we're kind of demonic. I might be a little scared to go."

When the possibility was raised of a dialogue between the two groups at a Wellness 2000 meeting (HLQ) there was a long silence followed by a number of people who argued that they saw nothing to be gained from such a dialogue. An HLQ activist said he thought that many CFC members were "the same types who join the NRA [National Rifle Association] and support right-wing militias." On the other hand, one of the leaders of CFC commented this way on their relationship to other alternative health networks,

> I would say the vast majority of the people [in the CFC] are conservative Christians. But people are comfortable at our meetings because we don't ostracize people because they're in the New Age movement but we don't want them bringing their crystals there and you know we're supporting our organization almost totally from Christian funding. But we don't want to kick these people out. We want to embrace them.

Later in the same interview, this CFC leader also commented on the resistance to New Age ideas from many of his friends who associated any interest in alternative health with New Age spirituality:

To the degree [New Age people] work in the Truth this is the degree that they'll have success. My friends say, "You're leaving the faith. You're crazy getting involved in this New Age crap. You know you got to stay away from that. They'll drag you into spirit guides and things of that sort."

In contrast to the conservative Christian belief system in the CFC, most of the participants in the holistic health network were quite alienated from institutionalized religion. One woman who was brought up as a Catholic but left the church, reflected on her experience:

I went back to the church a few times but I was disappointed because it was teaching a lot of fear- based things. What I learned in my Catholic studies was fear and guilt and I don't believe God is a punishing God for one second—or a judging God.

A traditional acupuncturist expressed a theme common among the members of the holistic health network: a rejection of the Christian concept of sin. She noted, "I never bought into the fact that we fell from grace with God. It didn't make sense to me. I believe we are born whole and radiant."

These cultural differences consist not only of clearly articulated contrasts between Christian and Eastern/metaphysical religious beliefs but are also embodied in the way meetings are run, leadership styles, and the way participants dress, talk, and interact with one another. In terms of leadership, the holistic health network, heavily influenced by the antibureaucratic ethos of 1960s radicalism, emphasizes democratic participation as well as group solidarity.[15] The leadership is quite self-effacing and wary of taking on too much responsibility. In contrast, the chiropractor who is the "figurehead" of the CFC exhibits some of the charisma and entrepreneurial zest found in evangelical Christian communities.

These differences would not be surprising to anyone. But of more interest are the similarities between the two networks, in terms of the beliefs of participants about conventional medicine and alternative health, personal freedom and government regulation, and a rejection of the excesses and lack of meaning in a consumer-oriented society. Moreover, we found some occasions in which members of the two networks interacted. Rather than emphasizing the differences, we were struck by the fact that alternative health is one of the few sites in which these two communities interact and share common allegiances and values.

The critique of the healthcare system articulated by CFC speakers and leaders is quite similar to that of holistic health participants. One CFC speaker put it this way,

> Healthcare reform props up a failing medical industry and a failing health care system . . . Probably everyone you know is sick. The medical system is not about healing; it is about cutting and drugging . . . The system focuses on symptoms and not causes . . . Why don't we hear [about low-tech, nontoxic, and inexpensive treatments for disease]? Because the drug companies can't make money from it.

Other CFC speakers have advocated a "cashless economy based on biblical principles of health" and railed against the vested interests of organized medicine and drug companies.

> I hate conspiracies. The only conspiracy I see is that everyone is protecting turf. They [the medical profession] are going to have to surrender some of their thought patterns. They're going to have to agree that what they've done in the past was not to the best interest of their patients but to keep organized medicine organized and the drug companies profits high.

Critiques of conventional medicine among the holistic health participants we interviewed reflected many of the same themes. One participant in the macrobiotic study group put it this way: "I think that Western medicine just looks at symptoms and sort of slaps a drug on it and says, 'There, maybe it won't hurt so much.' But it doesn't do a damn thing for the root of the problem. That really irritates me." One midwife explained,

> The health care system is a mess. It's still an illness-oriented system. It is not preventive health oriented and there are a lot of people being left out . . . It's a very pervasive problem and it's going to be very difficult to fix because the insurance industry, the hospital industry, the M.D. industries are very powerful and are going to fight to the death to keep their hold on the system the way it is.

A massage therapist expressed concern that health care reform would fall short of a full reevaluation of the system that she felt was needed. In this respect, her sentiments are widely shared in the CFC:

It seems as though [health care reform] is an opportunity to broaden our understanding of what health is, what wellness is . . . It seems as though what we're going to end up with again is another illness-based model with some sort of token bits of what they're calling "preventive care," which are very allopathic anyway, immunization, screening for certain kinds of cancer, and that's all very allopathic. We might have had a chance to even think about what it is to be well and have people, perhaps, have a little more choice or leeway in pursuing what they feel is wellness.

Beyond a common critique of the health care system, which reflects common values about what health care should be, we also found agreement about the dangers of government health care regulation and the importance of personal freedom. One health store owner and naturopath (who was worried about the FDA regulation of herbs and vitamins) told us,

Well, I trust the government just about as far as I can throw an elephant . . . You know what happened to our freedom of choice and our freedom of rights? It's very distressing to me because I don't feel we are hurting anybody. What about regulating the drugs that they put out? All their experimental drugs and people die—last year alone there were close to ninety thousand deaths due to prescription drugs.

A CFC leader expressed similar sentiments about government agencies preventing health consumers from seeking the care they desire:

It's the old story—buyer beware. If everyone knows buyer has to beware and there's no one up there protecting you or I then we're a little more cautious of everything. But we have the mistaken idea that someone up there is protecting us from all these bad things and that's where the problem is. The fox is in charge of the hen house.

The emphasis on the freedom of health care providers to practice outside of the allopathic system and the freedom of patients to seek the kind of care they want is closely connected to a shared interest in voluntarism and self-help rather than a bureaucratically administered state. One HLQ activist in the context of praising "intentional communities," sounded an often heard theme: "Sometimes liberals don't get it. People do not want a big government." A CFC member, who in all likelihood is more conservative on a host of issues compared to his

New Age colleagues, sounded a similar note: "Government should not be involved in activities that are the responsibility of families, churches, and individuals." In terms of colonization theory, participants in both networks voice concern over the loss of self-supervision and autonomy as a result of the extension of the administrative state and what Ivan Illich calls the "disabling professions."[16]

Another commonly heard view that unites participants in both networks is that in alternative health there is a commitment to health, to a somewhat demanding set of practices, and to continuous education ("taking responsibility for one's health"). One animal rights activist who has been a patient of a number of alternative practitioners asserted,

> There's a big difference between people who rely on doctors and all their drugs and everything else and people like us who want to take charge of our own lives, our own health, who want to take responsibility for it. That's what I see is the difference—the lazy ones, the ones who don't care, the ones who really don't have a respect for their bodies . . . I think that people like us have a profound respect for their bodies' capability to heal.

One CFC leader also emphasized the commitment required in alternative health:

> It's a lot easier to go to chemo [chemotherapy] once a month than to change your whole lifestyle. In the past, the medical establishment was saying that's all they had to do. "Submit yourself to the table; we'll put you under the knife, give you anesthesia and make it as comfortable for you as possible. That's all you need to do." So we're really going against the grain of society as far as this lack of discipline.

Even among participants in the CFC (people who are largely "Christian conservatives") alternative health seems to produce or reinforce a critique of our society that goes well beyond the sphere of health care. One CFC member said,

> We're a gluttonous society and as a result we've lost it as far as the family is concerned. We want the quick fix. We want the cocaine to feel good . . . You have to have that excess to get the monkey off your back.

This concern with a culture of self-indulgence and "excess" and with the effect this has on families and relationships was something we also heard quite often from participants in the holistic health network. Here is one example:

> People are spending so much time outside to make a dollar and there doesn't seem to be the connectedness in the home. For the people that I know, mom and dad are at work full-time. The kids are at the babysitter. It's a reality. To buy a house and the two cars, it takes that much money and it's a problem. I don't know quite what the answers are. Sometimes I think maybe people could be happy with a little less and that might help. But the media is constantly telling you that you need more and more and other people around you constantly having more—it's a hard thing to do.

One elderly NLG activist, who described herself as a "conservative Christian" expressed a similar concern about the corrosive effect of modern life on the family and what she calls "life values." "Life values" are the skills and wisdom about nutrition, gardening, cooking, and health care that women once had but that are now disappearing because of the fast-paced nature of the modern world.

> I don't know what can be done. I'm not very optimistic about things. Because with the breakdown of the family for one thing—the breakdown of not only family values but life values, people don't care anymore about these things. I mean the general run of people. Of course they have to get their meals on the fly, on the run with all these fast foods and so forth, what can they do? How many families would have the time to do what I do. None, practically, at least none that are out there working for a living.

These themes (that alternative health participants are resisting the lack of self-discipline, excessiveness, and passivity of a consumer-oriented society) constitute an important part of alternative health's collective identity. Here we see a clear construction of a moral boundary between alternative health and the outside world, as well as a source of solidarity among movement participants.

Finally, we found participants in both networks at a regional meeting of the National Health Federation held in Pittsburgh. Members of both networks had booths and attended workshops and lectures. The Christian-oriented and somewhat conservative sounding rhetoric of NHF leaders did not inhibit cooperation based on common interests. In addition to occasional NHF conventions, members of both networks interact sporadically at the co-op lecture series in Pittsburgh and at CFC meetings. Thus, alternative health seems to be one of the few sites where these contrasting cultures can, at least partially, cooperate.

This sense of emergent collective identity in both networks can best be understood as an innovative response to the colonization of the lifeworld. Both groups are responding to the bureaucratic regulation of health and illness and to the commodification of social life, which are understood as fundamental sources of chronic illness as well as a general loss of meaning and direction. Through bureaucratic interventions in health care people are deskilled and no longer in control of their own health, becoming clients of bureaucratic services. With respect to commodification, members of both networks express a more complex, if not contradictory stance. While criticizing the role of money in the operation of biomedicine and its connection to the pharmaceutical industry as well the industrialization of food production, many of them work as entrepreneurs and oppose national health insurance because they fear this might limit their economic independence. Alternative health is also a hothouse for small companies distributing new products that can be increasingly found in health food stores and promoted at health fairs. In short, there seems to be a greater resistance to bureaucratization than to commodification, which reflects wider cultural and social currents.

The Politics of Alternative Health

This partial critique of commodification and greater sensitivity to the dangers of bureaucratization illustrate the way alternative health crosses the traditional political divide between Left and Right. If the core of a left-wing perspective on politics involves the enlargement of the sphere of nonmarket relations, then both networks, independent of how they characterize themselves politically (as liberal or conservative) move in this direction half way. At the local co-op, activists self-consciously resist efforts to make the co-op into another supermarket and are apprehensive about this possibility. Indeed, the activist we interviewed enjoyed working in the co-op precisely because it was not exclusively concerned with efficiency, profit, and hierarchical work relations. Wellness 2000, during its earlier period, attempted to bring practitioners and patients together in mutual aid and support through voluntarism and bartering. The CFC provides free information and events while the NLG for a long period functioned as a food co-op for people living outside the Pittsburgh area. The CFC meetings were designed to develop networks of people who could help and support one another in the treatment of illness.

However, this process contradicts other tendencies going in a different direction. Both networks are emeshed to a significant degree in small commodity production and entrepreneurship. While in the holistic network entrepreneurship is practiced but not acknowledged, in the CFC it is both practiced and celebrated. Much of what actually occurs in both networks is the exchange of money for products and services. Moreover, in the CFC new products are continuously displayed and promoted as solutions to a wide range of illnesses. In fact, alternative health is a cottage industry for the emergence of a host of new companies including alternative health dotcoms. From this point of view opposition to the "medical-industrial complex"[17] expresses a conflict between a monopoly and an emerging entrepreneurial sector, a feature of capitalism from its very beginning.

The antibureaucratic ethos of alternative health is also consistent with elements of the Left as well as the conservative political traditions. The emphases on self-care and what we've called technologies of the self provide a strong antibureaucratic impulse rooted in the practical consciousness of everyday life. The "care of the self" provides the basis for a persistent and ongoing suspicion of expertise because it is bound up with ongoing concerns with health and illness. However, this antibureaucratic impulse may be taken up in different ways; on the Left the emphasis on prefigurative politics (the creation of new associations and communities that embodies a desired future)[18] and on the Right the glorification of the market and entrepreneurship. The central tendency in the holistic network is for the antibureaucratic impulse to be expressed through the conquest of new social, political, and cultural territories, the creation of new ways of living (such as intentional communities) and new associations (such as Wellness 2000 and HLQ). For the CFC and NLG, on the other hand, the antibureaucratic impulse is in large part expressed through a commitment to entrepreneurship and the market. But this valorization of the market is always embedded in some conception of an organic community and the values within which market relations operate. No member of the CFC would say that the purpose of life is buying and selling. Instead, buying and selling is a vehicle for the expression and perpetuation of a way of life that is religiously grounded.

The discourses that channel the care of the self in different directions can be understood by revisiting Offe's distinction between three levels of power and change in the modern world. If the reader will recall, these levels are: policymakers within the state and their shifting coalitions; social movements and interest groups who try to affect policy makers in different directions; and finally the "microsphere" of power, which involves everyday interactions and the unregulated flow of information, images, and ideas that circulate in the lifeworld. The care of the self has its shaping force within the microsphere of power. Here values and ideas concerning the person and her relation to the world, including nature, circulate. Within this sphere there is the basis for a cultural shift toward what some have called "postmaterial values,"[19] a noninstrumental view of the natural world, a critique of progress and the work ethic and the importance of extended and porous communities within which people from different backgrounds can mutually enrich one another. This value shift has experiential roots in the shared health practices of participants in both networks. This value shift ultimately must influence higher levels of decision making, even if this is gradual, piecemeal, and indirect.

The implications of this value shift depend on the way these values are transformed and mediated at the second level of power, where discourse and organization operate. Here, alternative health has a tendency to pressure policy makers in different ways. Conservatively oriented groups advocate the deregulation of the health care market and oppose any model of universal health care provided by the state. This view is consistent with the general dislike of the Keynesian regulatory state and its system of social provision. More progressively oriented groups are more open to regulation and universal health care provided it allows for choice of all health care protocols. The discourse that resists regulation is coupled with a defense of a traditional way of life, rooted in biblical values. For progressive groups, diversity and self-invention are embraced as cultural ideals. However, we shouldn't take these divisions too far at these higher levels of power. The value shift at the level of the lifeworld creates the possibility for a reconceptualization of progress and its costs. There are hints and suggestions of this as the language of sustainable social and economic development works its way into the debates of organizations, experts, and even policy makers.

At the level of discourse what unites both progressives and conservatives in alternative health is the absence of a class analysis of health and illness. While progress and its glorification of quantitative growth are criticized, the connection between capitalism, class deprivation, and sickness is occluded. It is well documented that there is a strong correlation between many chronic diseases and class location. The latest research shows a strong correlation between psychological and physical illness and the lack of autonomy and satisfaction of people at work. For example, over the past few years scores of studies have documented the relationship between social class, power, and illness. In fact, the research shows that class position and its attendant experience of status deprivation are better predictors of a wide range of chronic illnesses including heart disease, arthritis, diabetes, and some types of cancer than genetics, exposure to carcinogens, and even lifestyle choices.[20]

Yet in all wings of alternative health such an analysis lies outside of their holistic frame of reference. In this sense their holistic model is not so holistic. While it includes mind, body, and spirit and their interaction, it neglects the weight of the social world and its class divisions. This in turn reflects a wider lack of a class awareness in new social movements, which instead emphasize the roles of client, consumer, and citizen rather than worker as the principal forms of deprivation.[21] Ironically, this neglect of the social world and its effect on health and illness is shared by biomedicine. Biomedicine too abstracts from power and class relations in order to discover the etiology and cure of disease. In this sense, just as entrepreneurial and market models influence the practices and understanding of alternative health, so too the lack of awareness of class relations shapes their understanding of the source and solution to the problems of health and illness. What is mostly left in the discourse of alternative health is the sovereign individual and his own choices.

This emphasis on the sovereign individual and his own choices assumes that health is primarily a matter of the choices of consumers. In this way alternative health winds up being uncritical of the role of markets and their impact on health care provision. For instance, it may well be the case that a nonmarket system of health care would be more open to alternative health than a market-based system. On a national level a market-based system would tend to drive health toward the use of sophisticated technology, patentable pharmaceutical drugs, and overspecialization. Much of what makes alternative health unique is that it relies on natural remedies that are not patentable, it reduces the degree of medical expertise because of its logic of self-care, and finally it relies on low-tech interventions. Therefore, the commercial value of its practices and products is not comparable to biomedicine's. In short, alternative health's partial celebration of the market works against its capacity to achieve its full promise.

New Meanings and Identities

The valorization of the individual at the level of discourse repeatedly collides with ongoing practices that involve mutuality through dense networks of support, which lead to new understandings of the self. While the vast majority of the practitioners we talked to were committed to their own therapy, unlike other professionals they also saw themselves as part of a larger process of change and did not place much importance on the value of one therapy compared to another, even their own. Indeed, we were repeatedly told that part of the value of their practice was to encourage patients to seek out other practitioners and associations such as study groups, cooking classes, lectures, and sellers of organic food. Our research suggests that these two segments of the alternative health community (the holistic network and the Christian network) can be usefully understood as new social movement networks in Melucci's sense. They are submerged in everyday life rather than engaging in visible political activities that confront authorities. For participants in both alternative health networks, the focus is not primarily on strategic action—challenging social institutions in order to bring about specific changes—but instead on challenging cultural codes associated with professional expertise, illness, and health, as well as embodying alternative lifestyle practices. These networks are also laboratories for cultural experimentation with new authority patterns, new forms of organization, and new ideas.

For most of our informants their own illnesses were the entry points in a process that gradually enlarged their critical sensibilities. The process begins when a variety of elements of everyday life (food, cooking, expertise, the environment, former relationships, and friendships) become problematized. Quite literally, much of what is thought to be most "natural" in life is thrown open to question and reexamination. Even those who had political commitments before their entry into alternative health report that older dormant involvements became reactivated or enriched.

For this reason, we argue that alternative health has some unique properties that differentiate it from other new social movement networks. The chief difference is that in alternative health opposition to the system is embodied in a very literal sense. What one chooses to eat, how food is prepared, the time it takes to prepare and eat one's meals, and the experience and interpretation of health and illness are integral aspects of how modern men and women experience their everyday lives. In redefining these experiences and offering an alternative way of life that embodies (at least in part) new meanings, alternative health keeps alive an awareness of the deficiencies of modern institutions. Alternative health activities are one important ongoing practice that sustains a critique of the system and, unlike other oppositional practices, cannot be discarded because the body cannot be so easily co-opted, assimilated, and forgotten. Otherwise, illness will return.

Our interviews suggest that illness is the entry point for many into various alternative health sites. For some of the other people we interviewed it was not their own physical illness but a life crisis of some kind.[22] How do those who begin with an illness or a life crisis (or both) end up with a commitment to alternative health and, for many, an alternative way of life? What are the larger implications of this emerging commitment and way of life?

Many of our informants made a special effort to convey to us how much they valued the quality of the relationship they first experienced with their alternative practitioner, as well as their experiences in group settings—shopping at the co-op, study groups, and meetings. Through these relationships they made emotional investments that solidified a commitment not only to alternative health but to a critique of elements of modern societies. One patient who became an active participant in the network run by the macrobiotic counselor explained:

> Everybody [in the alternative health community] is so warm. It's nice to know there's something out there beside the regular rat race. I don't even go to the Giant Eagle [the major grocery store chain in Pittsburgh]. You go to the food co-op and there's just a different atmosphere . . . When I go to the store today I feel so overstimulated . . . People say they don't have time to cook at home but they have time to drive to the supermarket, shop, wait to be served, [and] drive home which takes just as much time as cooking at home.

A young patient who suffered from candidiasis became friends with the naturopath who helped to cure her and established a barter relationship with her. She later interpreted her illness as "an important turning point" in her life that convinced her that majoring in business to make her mother happy was not the way to go. She is now involved in ecology organizations—an involvement that grew out of her alternative health activities.

In addition to the new relationships formed by the alternative health participant, including the relationship with his/her practitioner, there is also the demanding practice itself (technologies of the self), which has implications for how people lead their everyday lives and even for their relationships with friends and loved ones. We have gone over some of this terrain already in our discussion of technologies of the self but it worth repeating because now we want to show its relation to social movements. Cooking foods at certain temperatures, employing proper food combinations, shopping for and eating only organic foods, using a juicer, cleansing the body through enemas and colonics and other elaborate programs, fasting, breathing exercises, and herbal remedies all require a stance well outside of the dominant view of the patient as a passive object of medical expertise.

In both networks, but especially the CFC, a patient, or simply someone who wants to stay healthy, must make a serious commitment. At numerous meetings, CFC participants were told that disease is a result of built-up toxicity that is years in the making—a result of poor eating habits and of a food industry that depletes the soil of nutrients and injects food with preservatives, antibiotics, and other substances. Toxicity also comes from the physical environment—from an atmosphere depleted of oxygen, from pollution, and so on. The recommended treatment for this built-up toxicity involves a combination of fresh organic vegetables and fruits (raw foods), juicing, vitamin and mineral supplements, colonics and colon cleansing, oxidation treatments, and a supportive family and community environment that encourages faith, persistence, and responsibility for one's health.

According to numerous CFC speakers and patient testimonials, when a patient's underlying problem is attacked by an alternative healing modality, symptoms usually worsen. These periods in which symptoms worsen are called, as mentioned earlier, "healing crises." One woman put it this way, "The worse you become through your healing schedules the better it is." "Worse" means an intensification of the very symptoms from which one seeks relief. It may also mean the appearance of certain illnesses that one was afflicted with in early childhood. The body, it is argued, has physical memories that linger in new forms. This may mean pain, insomnia, indigestion, or fatigue. As a result, it is important for patients to understand what is happening to them and to be involved actively in their own treatment. Otherwise, this peculiar path to recovery will not be sustained, especially since the logic of a healing crisis contradicts the immediate relief that conventional medicine promises and that even the wider culture demands as its ultimate goal. Moreover, healing crises require a depth of commitment from the patients' loved ones.

In the holistic health network, there is also an emphasis on healing and health as a demanding set of practices. One nurse, who does therapeutic touch as well as a range of other alternative modalities, explained that her approach to healing demands a lot from patients:

> This kind of work is not the magic bullet. It's not the easy way. The kind of work I do is teaching them how to tap into their own inner abilities for healing. That means they have to do the work. I can't do the work, and it's a road to transformation, it's a road to change that they will be different when they're done with this program than when they started. And those changes have to be made by them and sometimes it's difficult and some of it requires a lot of work, a lot of time, a lot of soul searching . . . No one can heal you, not me, not the doctor, not any external force. What we need to do is to take stock of what our habits are, what our thought patterns are, what our life patterns are, how we cope with life.

In short, patients undergoing alternative therapy (and most practitioners began as patients) cannot continue to live as they had before.

We have constructed, based on our interviews, an ideal type of a person who enters the alternative health community and adopts an alternative regimen. Such a participant experiences four sets of changes. Each change takes the person from the immediacy of everyday life to a connection with others and with larger issues, from illness as a private trouble to illness and health as social problems. With each transformation the person becomes increasingly committed to alternative health as a community and as a way of life.

First, as a person forms a relationship with an alternative practitioner and begins a healing regimen, he/she acquires a critical vantage point or "generalized other" within which he/she can evaluate former (and at times present) relationships with doctors. A number of patients said they were told by their M.D.s that they had psychological problems or that it was "all in your head" when their symptoms did not fit accepted diagnostic categories. One activist subsequently linked this kind of treatment to "our male-dominated medical profession" who "treat women as guinea pigs." Another woman with severe allergies remembered that her family doctor discounted her rashes and headaches and told her mother to "take her to the shrink." "That sort of turned me against doctors right there. What an ego on this man— because he couldn't find the problem, it was all in my mind." Other people complained about being given drugs after only a five-minute session. One patient with Crohn's disease told us that as a result of her experiences with alternative health she relates to her conventional doctor differently:

> I am always questioning my doctor because she or he will always rec-ommend certain tests and medication. I am always questioning, "Is this necessary or is this medication necessary?" And we just kind of negotiate back and forth.

Second, as this process unfolds, friends and loved ones must get used to the person's new eating habits, health regimen, and lifestyle, which at times produces conflict and uneasiness. This conflict impresses upon the person a sense that he/she is "different" and may also lead to a strengthening of convictions about the value of alter-native health. One woman commented on the typical reactions of others to a person who becomes committed to alternative health:

> People see changes in their friends and then they ask questions. People say, "My husband thinks I'm crazy. . . ." They turn up their noses when I get my lunch out. You know it all changes. It all hap-pened to me when I got started. They thought I was crazy and made fun of me. You have to keep a sense of humor about it and you have to keep your convictions and keep in mind why you're doing it.

Another woman whose involvement began just a few years ago said that her friends were not interested in alternative health, "so I've learned to make new friends." For another patient and now alternative health advocate, her friends just had to accept her new lifestyle:

> They [her friends] have no choice but to recognize that I'm a little dif-ferent now. When I show up for a week or two to visit my friends in Kansas City or to go home for a couple of weeks and I arrive with my box of food and my pressure cooker and like, "Oh God, she's moving in with all her weird food again. Make room on the kitchen counter" [laughter].

Third, as the person begins to branch out from his/her first rela-tionship with an alternative practitioner in order to associate with others who also think of themselves as "different," an identification develops with an alternative health community. A growing immersion in the dense world of co-op shopping, study groups, expos, cooking classes, lectures, and patient testimonials begins to produce a sense of "we," an identification with a community that rests on a considerable investment of time, energy, emotion, money, and new friendships. Identification with alternative health is not simply a "belief" but is rooted in an emerging way of life. Collective identity, a sense of "we"—the creation of boundaries and solidarities—doesn't flow automatically from structural location or from discontent.

Fourth, as the person interacts with members of this community, who come from diverse backgrounds and who often have experiences in other social movements, new value commitments emerge. Approximately one-third of our informants called themselves "feminists" (two said they were "pro-life feminists") and said that alternative health was the source of their commitment to the empowerment of women. A few also said that they were critical of the "cult of victimization" that they associated with some versions of feminism (and the recovery movement) but still retained a feminist commitment.

Perhaps the clearest political stance that flows out of involvement in alternative health is a commitment to ecology. Once a person begins to be committed to organic food, he/she often becomes aware of modern agricultural practices, which in turn may lead to an awareness of other ecological issues. One NLG activist who describes herself as "culturally conservative" has, as a result of her years in alternative health, become an ecology activist. Her involvement in forming an organic food co-op in the mid 1950s led to contacts and associations with groups outside of her community. She became active in the Western Pennsylvania Solar Energy Society and still teaches a course at a local community college on "Living Better for Less." While supporting traditional family values, her health activism led to new political involvements. She is "enthusiastic" about Ralph Nader, thinks "he is on the right track," and likes the idea of "breaking up the two party system." In addition to changing the health care system to allow people more freedom she also believes that we need to "change the whole way we produce food."

In addition, we have found connections between alternative health and animal rights activism[23] as well as commitment to peace issues. The attention that alternative practitioners have paid to the AIDS crisis may be providing a route for gay patients to connect with gay rights networks. Two of the practitioners we interviewed treat AIDS patients and are themselves active in gay and lesbian organizations. While we are not claiming that all activists in the feminist health movement, ecology, gay rights, animal rights, and peace networks begin in alternative health, we are suggesting that participants in alternative health come into contact with diverse movement beliefs and networks. In some cases this stimulates new commitments and involvements. As one co-op shopper told us, "Most of the alternative thinking people are into alternative food. The main connection between progressive communities is food."[24]

In all of this networking what is striking is the central role of women. As we have mentioned the vast majority of the patients and practitioners in the alternative health networks we've studied are women. Why is this so and what is its significance? Obvious explanations come to mind; the association of women with healing, helping, and caring as well the career opportunities available in a less male-dominated sector of the health care industry. More interestingly, we suggest that women are more likely than men to be the vehicles through which traditions, including natural remedies, are kept alive and passed on through the generations. Our interviews support this point as many women told us about how they learned about herbs and other remedies from their mothers and grandmothers. Such a stance as custodians of tradition and natural remedies can lead to skepticism toward male dominated medical expertise and its high-tech interventions. In this sense women may be open to healing traditions that evoke intergenerational bonds between women and connections to the "natural" world. In this respect, women in both networks tend to see themselves as protectors of a noncommodified and nonbureaucratic domain of practices.

The three levels of power we've identified previously have embedded within them an interesting feminist subtext. The experiences of mutuality and support, respect for traditions and valorization of the natural operate within the microsphere of everyday life or what we have called previously the "weak public sphere." It is within this sphere where some women have predominant influence. We might even go so far as to argue that technologies of the self constitute a gendered practice. However, these impulses at the base become redirected and attenuated at higher levels of power, which are more male-dominated.[25] At these levels, models of possessive individualism become more predominant. The slogan, "The individual is responsible for his health," can mean that individuals are blamed for their illness and held exclusively accountable for maintaining their health. Alternative health becomes in this sense oriented more toward the market and entrepreneurial activity. The network character of health care is weakened, which is the level where women's influence is greatest.

Alternative Health as a New Social Movement

We argue that alternative health can be understood as a new social movement for the following reasons. First, it is anchored in large part in experiences outside the sphere of production. Chronic disease, while closely related to positions within the economy, is also a conse- quence of global factors that affect everyone—pollution, devitalized foods, and the speeding up of life as people adapt to a new interna- tional system of economic production. These experiences provide the basis for alliances and networks outside the sphere of work. Second, these experiences provide opportunities for people to enter into rela- tionships within the weak public sphere and therefore constitute sub- merged networks within the microsphere of power. Third, these submerged networks connect to the larger world through a common resistance to bureaucratization and to a lesser extent commodification. What's unique about alternative health's submerged networks is that they are rooted in persistent health problems and register in bodily terms the costs of capitalist modernization. Precisely because of its bodily practices, alternative health opens people in a persistent way to submerged networks in other movements that have more articulated organizational forms, all of which have a bearing indirectly on health and illness.

The health practices we have described are efforts to set limits on a central tendency in modern societies—the absorption by the "media of money and power" of practices and knowledge that had rested in fam- ilies, communities, and in public spheres. The medical-industrial complex is a leading instrument of colonization and resistance to it is coming from the Christian Right as well as elements of the cultural Left. For both, healing must somehow reconnect with the active knowledge that people bring into their everyday lives and that emerges from the lifeworld.

Another implication of our analysis is the importance of a movement's relationship to everyday life. One explanation of the ability of some movements to resist absorption (co-optation) is the extent to which it has solid roots in submerged networks, which is in some sense independent of the movement's organizational dimension. Alternative health, while lacking organization and resources, generates and sustains oppositional and alternative meanings because its sub- merged networks are so uniquely embedded in everyday life. Finally, alternative health may be the place where we can find the most ongoing basis for a value shift in the structures of everyday life in modern societies. This is why people who are in the New Age, are hippies, work in co-ops, are feminists, and are Christian fundamentalists—and many in between—share, in potential, this common site and find themselves together on this terrain.

If it is true that alternative health is implicated in a fundamental value shift the question becomes, How is it sustained or altered when it becomes partially integrated into the dominant health care system? How does alternative health transform institutions and how is alternative health transformed as a result of this process?

CHAPTER 6

From Alternative
to Complementary Medicine

Social movements can be understood as existing in a tension between an institutional level and what Melucci calls a movement's "submerged networks."[1] Submerged networks are "cultural laboratories," largely invisible since they are embedded in everyday life. Individuals move in and out of these networks, rather than being totally committed to them. In this arena, similar to aspects of what Habermas calls the "lifeworld," there are flows of images, information, and ideas that can be a source of creativity for a movement.[2] The drying up of these subcultural roots may be as detrimental to a movement as the failure to make itself visible through ongoing political action and through processes of institutionalization. However, if a movement only exists as a submerged network, the danger is marginalization. In other words, the movement loses touch with the institutional direction of society as a whole. This results in two consequences; the movement, through "cooptation," loses its capacity to challenge power holders and, on the other hand, as isolated and marginal, it may develop conspiratorial fantasies and delusions about its own omnipotence. Therefore, we argue, the power of any movement requires a creative tension between its submerged and institutional dimensions. In short, it must become what we call a "dual movement."[3]

The idea of a dual movement was suggested to us by our previous discussion of how expert cultures mediate knowledge with everyday actors in the lifeworld. We discovered that successful mediation requires

155

the mutual transformation of experts and everyday actors while at the same time the differences between the two do not totally collapse. This symbiosis and separation of the two are critical for their mutual enrichment. Without this mediation, people become alienated from their own bodies and from the larger world around them. Experts, as a result, lose any sense of connection between their technical knowledge and its significance in terms of the larger world around them.

Alternative Health's Institutionalization

With this in mind, we explore in this chapter the growing institutionalization or "integration" of alternative health and how this bears on the capacity of alternative health to remain a dual movement. It's been approximately eight years since armed FDA agents raided Dr. Jonathan Wright's clinic, then president of the National Health Federation and prominent holistic M.D. They confiscated bags of vitamins but found no illegal substances. Also during this period the FDA proposed to regulate herbs and vitamins as drugs, a proposal that could not withstand the opposition of pro–alternative health congressmen, both Republicans and Democrats. At a NHF convention held a few years later, speaker after speaker spoke out against federal government repression of the alternative health community and saw this as an expression of an overly intrusive, if not repressive state. Of course, the alternative health community is broader than the NHF but during this period there was a widely held suspicion, not only of the medical-industrial complex—the close links between the medical profession, hospitals, pharmaceutical, and health insurance companies but of the administrative state, which made the practice of alternative medicine by practitioners and patients difficult.

Much has changed in a relatively short period of time. David Eisenberg's now famous surveys documented the widespread popularity of alternative health products and services. Largely positive media coverage has also contributed to and reflected this widespread interest. In addition, the National Institutes of Health (NIH) created an Office of Alternative Medicine (now the Center for Complementary and Alternative Medicine) which now has a sixty-nine million-dollar budget to research the effectiveness of alternative health modalities. In 1996, the OAM provided the funding for a research center at Bastyr University, which, as a result, became the nation's first publicly funded naturopathic center of medicine. It should also be noted that past and present OAM directors have forcefully lobbied for alternative health to be integrated into dominant health care system and recommended rigorous scientific testing of alternative health modalities. Today, 64 percent of U.S. medical schools have at least one course on alternative medicine,[4] research institutes and schools specializing in non-allopathic approaches exist throughout the country, health insurance companies are beginning to cover some alternative health protocols, especially for heart disease, and many hospitals are opening up complementary medicine clinics. In short, developments within the state and in the "medical industrial complex" have created new political opportunities[5] for the alternative health movement to enhance its professional status and establish closer links to conventional medicine.

What are we to make of all of this? The answer seems simple. Alternative medicine is nowhere near as marginalized as it once was. Practitioners and health storeowners fear the FDA less while they sell more of their products and services. Inroads in medical school curricula and new complementary medicine clinics create the potential for a mutual enrichment of both conventional and alternative medicine. But in light of the earlier analysis of alternative health's dual movement character, the stakes involved in the process of this growing institutionalization are far more complex. Is this success coming at the price of the vitality of alternative health's submerged networks and core identity? Is the health care system changing to accommodate the demands of a popular health movement or is the movement accommodating to the requirements of the system? If the former is the case then we have an instance of successful institutionalization. If the latter is the case, the movement loses its creative base and dual character.

A good way to explore these issues is to look at what actually happens when holistic M.D.s and health care practitioners work within the institutional setting of biomedicine. What tensions exist within the alternative health community—between the holistic doctors and practitioners that work within more institutionalized settings and those who remain embedded in its submerged networks? In order to answer these questions we studied a complementary medicine clinic at a prominent hospital. These clinics are becoming quite common throughout the country and are an ideal setting in which to examine the question of the compatibility of alternative medicine and the dominant health care system. Clinic directors as well as doctors and practitioners associated with these clinics must engage in a delicate balance between preserving the core of alternative or "complementary" medicine but also accommodating to the institutional demands of hospitals—the core of the conventional health care system. The clinic in Pittsburgh exists in the largest hospital chain in the city and one of the largest in the country. All of the features of modern medicine against which alternative health has organized can be found there—highly specialized medical expertise, sophisticated medical technology, and complex bureaucratic rules and procedures, and the pressure to generate income.

The Complementary Medicine Clinic

In the spring of 1997 a nurse practitioner, with the help of another nurse who had already been practicing therapeutic touch at the hospital, a sympathetic psychiatrist, and a few others, approached the chief of the department of medicine with a proposal to form a complementary medicine clinic. These clinics were already in place in many hospitals and the Eisenberg article published in the *New England Journal of Medicine* in 1993 had given alternative medicine some degree of legitimacy. With some in-house funding and the fortuitous hiring of a prominent holistic physician from another city, the clinic opened a year later. In addition, members of the hospital's board of directors supported the clinic because of personal experiences with alternative medicine.

The clinic now occupies a suit of offices where three holistic physicians, one psychiatrist, and fifteen practitioners offer patients a wide range of alternative health therapies—natural remedies such as botanical medicine, naturopathic counseling, and nutritional medicine; mind-body approaches such as biofeedback, EMDR (eye movement desensitization and reprocessing), relaxation therapies, and guided imagery; and finally, bodywork therapies such as acupuncture, shiatsu, and therapeutic massage. The clinic also offers wellness classes in yoga, therapeutic touch, massage therapy, and meditation. Patients are required to have a physician referral to obtain any of the health services at the clinic. Since there are three M.D.s on the staff this is not a problem although the fact that few patients come with a referral from their own doctors is significant. Any new therapy that a practitioner or M.D. wants to introduce must be approved by the hospital, and the clinic's steering committee meets with members of the hospital administration on a weekly basis. Hardly any patient has insurance coverage for alternative therapies, so that payments are out of pocket.

Interviews with the administrative, program, and medical directors of the center shed some light on the motivations of the hospital for agreeing to open the clinic but this is still shrouded in mystery. While cautioning us that she was not "privy to the inner thoughts of the administration," the clinical director believes that the clinic creates a "warm and fuzzy feeling" for the hospital, and can provide the hospital with some positive publicity. At any rate, the work done at the clinic is thought to be "harmless." At the same time, the clinic is under increasing pressure to produce academically credible research to justify their clinical practices and to prove to the business side of the hospital that the clinic can be financially stable and self-sufficient within a few years. As we will see, there are good reasons to question whether either can be achieved without considerable cost to the core identity of alternative medicine. Another, perhaps critical element is the fact that, as mentioned earlier, certain members of the hospital board of directors had family members whose chronic conditions were helped by alternative medicine.

The medical director sees the origins of the center as an accident; there were people "with vision" who had an influence on the hospital administration who then "let it happen" without really understanding what they were doing. After it started, the clinic grew in terms of public awareness, patients treated, and the number of practitioners employed by the clinic, so that now it has become "sort of an embarrassing baby to take care of but you couldn't drop it at this point." Why are complementary medicine clinics opening throughout the country? The medical director believes that there is a lot of NIH research money available (sixty million dollars) and to get a piece of this you need patients and a clinic that will attract them so that you can establish research protocols. The other is a marketing motivation. The hope is that through advertising their complementary clinics, hospitals can appeal to a wider segment of the medical market.

According to an internal study of clinic patients, 75 percent are women between forty-five and sixty, and 5 percent racial minorities. Patients tend to be middle to upper middle class since treatments are not covered by insurance. Most patients suffer from chronic illnesses that don't respond well to conventional medicine. Fifteen percent of patients suffer from arthritis, 15 percent from migraines, 10 percent from cancer, 8 percent from heart disease, 13 percent from depression and anxiety, and another 13 percent from irritable bowel and other intestinal disorders. All of these problems, according to the medical director, "have a huge mental component."

Beyond this demographic and medical profile, it appears that patients who come to the clinic have one of two approaches to conventional medicine. They have either exhausted the therapies offered by conventional medicine (usually chronic pain and terminally ill patients) and are coming to the clinic as a last resort, or "want the best of both worlds." These patients, who are often oncology patients who have just been diagnosed, are well educated about alternative cancer treatments and are trying to devise a treatment regime that will combine chemotherapy and alternative approaches that emphasize building up the immune system.

The Patient-Practitioner Relationship at the Clinic

To what extent is the patient-practitioner relationship at the clinic a departure from the dominant model? The approach of the clinic to their patients is somewhat pragmatic. They have a range of innovative programs, which are available for patients who are comfortable with approaches that depart from the medical model. But at the same time they are willing to provide alternative treatments that don't require a lot of time and patient effort. As one clinic practitioner put it,

> Some patients come here at different levels so you have to approach them on their level. Some just want a pill you know . . . something that you do and it should have an outcome frequently. It's not a transformative process for them. And that's fine. We do that. But the people who want to go beyond that, we introduce them to people who will help them go on in that direction.

The medical director of the clinic, though, is uncomfortable with the tendency to "give patients what they want" even while recognizing the economic pressures to process patients. He worries that

> it would be very easy to corrupt alternative practitioners and the way it would happen is that what will be squeezed out is the part that takes time. One of the most important is mind-body medicine. It doesn't happen in a ten-minute visit. But some things can happen quickly like acupuncture needles—you can have fifteen rooms and we have practitioners who do that. You can sell supplements and herbs without any interaction with a patient just like you'd prescribe medicine. These are the approaches that will actually take over.

While these pressures exist, the practitioner-patient relationship does depart from the dominant model in a number of ways. All three directors of the clinic commented on something they called the "patient culture" or the "waiting room culture." One practitioner saw this as the key to the success of the clinic.

> When people enter here they enter a culture, and we might try one intervention but that's not what really changes people, it's that they now have entered a culture and they talk to other people and suddenly have a whole window on a new world and they start entering that world and trying different things and it's that experience that ultimately leads people into a healing path. Which door they go through is really not that important, whether they try massage or acupuncture or biofeedback or whatever. Once they buy into it they evolve and that's the process that brings upon a transformation.

According to another holistic physician at the clinic who is doing a study of the effect of reiki (a form of energy medicine similar to therapeutic touch) on asthma patients, the waiting room culture creates a kind of synergy that makes it difficult to determine why patients do better when they do.

> There's this little study I'm doing about asthma and reiki and I found that after the fourth or fifth treatment that patients were doing multiple therapies without telling anyone because they're socialized by this waiting room culture. They do vitamin shopping with other patients, comparing notes on herbs, etcetera.

Everyone we interviewed mentioned the existence of this "patient culture" or "waiting room culture." Indeed, the program director saw this culture as the main reason for the clinic's existence.

> That's the struggle with integrating something like this with a mainstream medical center. It's that the assumptions by which you run outpatient clinics in conventional medicine don't apply here because the assumptions are individualizing and they deny a patient culture and what we're actually about is to create a patient culture that then heals itself. We're sort of the vehicle whereby the culture emerges and operates. For instance we've had a lot of trouble because our administrator doesn't want patients wandering through the hallways and going into the coffee room and coming in here and just hanging out. But that's what our patients expect to be able to do. They expect to be able to come in and wander the halls and get coffee because that's the model of medicine they want.

The clinic has a range of patient programs that go well beyond the one on one encounter of doctor and patient found in biomedicine. For example, the clinic runs an asthma study group where patients practice meditation or guided imagery and talk to one another about various aspects of complementary medicine that seem to work for them. So it's not clear when they do show improvement whether it's the meditation or guided imagery or all the other modalities they have been exposed to in this group setting. Moreover, the social support and encouragement received from other patients may also have a therapeutic effect. There is a wealth of clinical evidence not only about mind-body effects in healing but also the therapeutic value of social support for certain categories of patients.

Here is certainly a process that departs from the medical model of the doctor as expert and the patient as a diseased body occupying a "sick role." Moreover, it is hard to imagine a patient culture in conventional medicine, at least not the type described here. Other doctors and practitioners described a similar process. One used the word *synergy* to account for the way patients learn from one another and then incorporate more alternative therapies into their lives. Needless to say, in this environment, when there are results, it is hard to isolate one factor that is responsible.

One of the more innovative programs at the center is something called a "healing intensive." The former program director, Dr. Madrona, is the originator of this program. In the healing intensive patients undergo an intensive experience modeled after Native American healing rituals and philosophies. Patients receive two to seven hours per day of therapeutic attention including journal writing and discussion of what they've written, group discussions with other patients, hypnosis, body therapy, acupuncture, therapeutic touch, cognitive-behavioral therapy, family therapy, projective techniques including the use of Native American images, shields, or animal images, and ceremony. The intensive concludes on the seventh evening with a sweat lodge ceremony. All throughout this process patients receive guidance from mentors and coaches who "help them to focus on themselves and have a spiritual journey."

Clearly, this approach is not for everyone, but for those who have experienced it, the clinic has received rave reviews. Patients leave the week-long process feeling as though their "illness was a teacher" and experiencing fewer symptoms and reduced pain. A number of terminally ill cancer patients experienced a full remission of their cancer. One of these patients wrote about her experiences in a *Ladies Home Journal* article.

While none of the 105 patients who have been through a healing intensive complained, the program director who started this program has come under attack from a number of physicians in the hospital— in part because of these healing intensives and their use of Native American ceremonies. The program director has resigned under pressure, despite the fact that it was his reputation and innovative programming that resulted in the growth of the clinic. Currently (as of May 2000), according to Jane Dufield (*Pittsburgh Post-Gazette*), a spokeswoman for the hospital, "The investigation into all aspects of alternative medicine [at the hospital] is continuing. Until the study is complete, [the hospital] can't specifically say what the future holds for the [complementary medicine clinic]."

It appears that fundamentally challenging the dominant medical model has its costs. Despite internal records that show that 65 percent of clinic patients report a significant improvement in their condition after treatment at the center, and despite mounting scientific evidence for mind-body effects in illness and healing,[6] opposition to the center from physicians remains strong. Yet pressures come from patients as well, although of a very different kind. One holistic doctor at the clinic remarked with a little tongue in cheek that patients are too assertive and knowledgeable. That is irritating

> because they are telling you what the treatment should be and you feel a little straightjacketed. Sometimes that's not good because you're the doctor. They do need expert advice. It's good for them to be informed and ask questions but they should be open to getting help from another human being. Sometimes we're [the doctors] the ones who feel like machines.

So some practitioners at the clinic feel pulled between the hospital that would like them to adopt a conventional model of medical expertise and stay away from controversial approaches that involve patients, and their more knowledgeable patients who challenge any notion of medical expertise.

Evaluating Alternative Health Protocols

Another significant tension at the clinic and one that reflects a larger issue in alternative medicine is the pressure to conduct clinical research to demonstrate the efficacy of alternative treatment modalities. All the directors and physicians we talked to believed that this was "trying to fit a round peg into a square hole," although they are making an effort to conduct the double blind studies that fit the biomedical model of research. The dominant research model calls for clinical trials whose goal is to determine the relationship between a particular therapeutic intervention and a specific outcome. The problem is that the more alternative/complementary medicine retains its identity, the less it is possible to disentangle one therapy from another or for that matter a therapeutic intervention from the personal relationships between practitioners and other patients that are always part of the healing process. In contrast to the disdain for the "placebo effect" in conventional medicine, proponents of alternative medicine argue that the placebo effect demonstrates "that the body has the ability to heal itself under the right belief system if you tap into that belief system." In other words, activating the placebo effect is part of what alternative medicine is trying to do while at the same time intervening in other ways—through herbs, vitamins, massage, acupuncture needles, organic food, among other things.

Two of the physicians at the center recently had a grant proposal rejected by the NIH because there were too many variables under study. The research design compared a holistic program for fibromialga (a form of arthritis that conventional medicine has not had any success with) with conventional treatment. The holistic program included meditation, reiki, guided imagery, and cognitive restructuring. Patients would be encouraged to exercise and change their diet. Herbs would be available but the selection and amount would vary from patient to patient. The degree to which patients would be exposed to reiki and therapeutic touch (forms of "energy medicine") would also depend on the personality of patients since what patients think will help them is a significant part of the self-healing process. Encouraging patient involvement in devising a treatment regime is also essential to the holistic approach in alternative medicine. The NIH reviewers of the proposal rejected it because the research design included too many modalities, so that it would be impossible to determine which intervention produced positive results. The PIs responded to these criticisms by asking why it was so important to isolate one factor—at this early stage. If it could be demonstrated that a holistic regime worked better than a conventional one wouldn't that be step forward? The issue here is a serious one. In the United States more than other countries, it is not enough to demonstrate the effectiveness of a program of interventions in treating patients if you can't demonstrate a cause and effect relationship between a specific variable and a specified outcome.

The fact that no money is available for complementary medicine clinics to engage in clinical research that doesn't fit the biomedical research model—double blind, randomized studies—puts these clinics in a bind. If they try to demonstrate that a particular modality has therapeutic effects, they know they will have very limited success since this means treating alternative medicine nonholistically. But if they try to design a study to demonstrate the effectiveness of a holistic program of interventions, an approach that comes close to reflecting the philosophy of alternative medicine, no one will fund it.

The Submerged Networks and the Clinic

The biographical consequences for doctors and practitioners who work in this setting departs somewhat from the typical pattern you find among practitioners in the subculture—most of whom have their own practice or own their own stores. Most of the practitioners we interviewed who have their own practice described their entry into alternative medicine as something similar to a religious conversion experience. Many were disenchanted with former careers, had experienced divorces, were victims of domestic violence or had serious illnesses themselves. Alternative medicine represented a new way of living and for practitioners a career that offered a significant amount of autonomy and creativity. But for the physicians and practitioners at the clinic we heard a different story. The administrative director, a nurse practitioner, said that there is a delicate balance between maintaining a holistic lifestyle and keeping up with the stresses and pressures of working in the clinic. In other words, she said, it's difficult at the clinic to practice what you preach. Work-related stress is common among professionals but most alternative health practitioners we interviewed outside the clinic saw their work as integrated in a balanced way into their lives. Typically, their entry into alternative medicine was an escape from a former lifestyle that sacrificed health and personal growth to career advancement.

We also wanted to find out how practitioners at the clinic related to the broader alternative health subculture and what members of the subculture thought of the clinic. We tried contacting people—both alternative health practitioners, activists, and patients we had interviewed over the past few years—and their responses were mixed. Many saw the clinic as evidence of alternative health's success and were proud of this achievement. But at the same time many were skeptical that alternative medicine could flourish in this setting. Among the proponents of cleansing regimes using herbs, minerals, and natural foods the view is that conventional drug-based therapy is fundamentally incompatible with their purposes. In fact, the goal of "detoxification" is to in part remove the effects of drugs. In this corner of the alternative health subculture, there is no way for alternative and conventional medicine to coexist.

Among the practitioners in the clinic there was an ambivalent stance toward the broader subculture. The program director at the clinic characterized alternative health activists as "groupie types" and thought that most patients at the clinic had little association with the subculture although they were quite knowledgeable about alternative health approaches to their own illnesses. The "waiting room" and patient culture she described at the clinic seemed to be something quite distinct from the broader subculture of co-op shopping, lectures, study groups, health fairs, cooking classes, and the like. On the other hand, one of the holistic physicians who practices at the clinic also has an office with two massage therapists in a nearby neighborhood. Her identity is more closely associated with ongoing alternative health activities in the local area. She is skeptical about the long-term viability of the clinic because of all the obstacles the hospital administration is placing in its path.

While the analysis presented here points to serious problems of incorporating alternative medicine into a hospital setting, a number of practitioners and holistic physicians told us there are advantages. The chief one is the discipline of having to explain and justify yourself to people who review what you're doing. While quite frustrating at times, the medical director considers it a "healthy process." Record keeping, clinical research, the credentializing and licensing process for practitioners gives the clinic credibility with patients and makes it possible for the clinic leadership to learn from past practices. This systematic learning process as well as the collaboration between a wide range of practitioners and physicians has resulted in some innovative programs—primarily the use of study groups and healing intensives, which incorporate social support, information sharing, and various therapeutic interventions into a comprehensive holistic approach to treating chronic disease. The hospital setting itself gives alternative medicine credibility and there is a subgroup of clinic patients who would not have seen an alternative practitioner outside of this setting.

Two Clinic Patients

In order to illustrate the benefits and liabilities of institutionalization we present two examples of patients who spent a considerable amount of time at the clinic. These people are representative of clinic patients in terms of gender, age, and level of education. In addition, problems of "multiple chemical sensitivity" and severe pain are examples of two common problems that patients who come to the clinic manifest. Moreover, these problems are difficult for conventional medicine to treat, which is typical for the larger group of clinic patients.

Aime Bartell describes her condition prior to her trip to Greece in 1993 as "high energy, and in good health," which supported a "high achieving" career and lifestyle. In Greece she was exposed to high levels of air pollution and on a nearby island to high levels of silicon from the sand. Upon her return, her office was in the process of being renovated. These three "toxic" exposures sparked a serious allergic reaction. As she put it, "I got allergies to everything." As a result she experienced continuous "migraine headaches." This connection, however, between her headaches and these three toxic exposures came from her holistic physician, Dr.Madrona, who diagnosed her illness as "multiple chemical sensitivity" (conventional medicine rejects this diagnostic category as did Mrs. Bartell's allergist). At work, in order to function she had to hold an ice pack on her head continuously. She worked with small children and they got used to seeing her with the ice pack and would laugh and say, "Mrs. Bartell has a headache today, can I feel your ice pack."

Her treatment began with an allergist who gave her a series of shots. She then saw a neurologist who prescribed pain medications all the while giving her MRIs and CT scans to determine the cause of her condition. She also saw a psychologist who taught her biofeedback and other pain relief techniques. Eventually she entered a pain clinic in another city where "stronger medicine" was prescribed. Despite all of these efforts, "the more medicine I took the sicker I got." Finally, her allergist, exasperated at his lack of success, told her about a "Native American" doctor who worked at the complementary medicine clinic. While undergoing conventional medical treatment she described herself as a "highly motivated patient" who would "stand on her head, if told by her doctors." Therefore, she listened to her allergist's advice and visited the clinic.

At the clinic she met Dr. Madrona who thought that since Aime had undergone conventional treatment without success and the tests did not show any known biochemical cause, she was a good candidate for a healing intensive. She was excited to get started because she looked forward to getting off all her medications, especially after reading about their toxic effect on the liver and kidneys. But, what caused her some anxiety about this entire process is that elements of it contradicted her own Christian religious background. Beyond her religious traditionalism, her family was also conventional in most other ways, so there was little preparation for this experience. As a "devout Christian" the thought of going through a sweat lodge "blew my mind," and, "I thought to myself how did my allergist get me into this situation." She did not participate in the sweat lodge because it "was not for her" but recognized its potential value for others.

But nevertheless, out of curiosity and desperation she went through with the overall healing intensive. She stayed at a local hotel, did not watch TV, and went to the clinic eight hours a day for an entire week. Each day she would see a range of practitioners and physicians who introduced her to a variety of modalities including guided imagery, stories and folk tales for therapeutic purposes, relaxation techniques and acupuncture, massage, yoga, EMDR, and cognitive restructuring to help her handle stress. She has participated in group events where stories were told and people reacted to the stories in terms of their own experiences and medical condition. She found this helpful because she realized she was not alone in experiencing severe pain and that these people grew to care about her. She learned, among other things, "that I have some control over the pain because they taught me techniques that allowed me to raise or lower the pain."

What really made a difference was the intravenous vitamin treatment she received. This treatment was classified as "experimental" and the clinic had to get approval from the hospital. Dr. Madrona initially wanted to administer higher dosages but this was rejected. Nevertheless, Mrs. Bartell made rapid progress after receiving this treatment. She kept a "pain journal" in which she would classify the level of pain each day through the use of colors and numbers and then would write about her experiences. During 1998, the year she started at the clinic, her "bad days" in terms of pain fell dramatically, so that by December 1998, twenty-seven out of thirty-one days were described as comprising low and tolerable levels of pain. Mrs. Bartell got the idea of writing a journal from Dr. Madrona's Native American stories. She still calls upon many of the images (in this case snakes, a blue mountain that embodies the destination of health, among other things) that were suggested in these stories to help her make sense of her illness and give her hope for recovery. In her pain journal, she draws pictures to illustrate her daily experiences and comments on these pictures.

As mentioned earlier, Dr. Madrona diagnosed her illness as multiple chemical sensitivity. This was discovered when she went into shock from an antibiotic treatment for bronchitis and received high dosages of steroids, which surprisingly eliminated her "migraine headaches." Madrona realized that steroids are not an effective treatment for migraines and therefore her problem must be elsewhere. This led to her successful treatment by intravenous vitamins. Her allergist, nevertheless, resisted this diagnosis as a "faddish" product of a California subculture (Madrona is from California). This collision between the world of alternative and conventional medicine caused her much distress and anxiety since she wished to maintain access to both. She therefore wanted both doctors to talk it through and work it out with each other, which they eventually did. Eventually, her allergist admitted that her improvement was remarkable but could not explain it. Unfortunately, since undergoing alternative treatment she had to pay out of pocket, a considerable cost. This has forced her to cut back on her treatment and her condition has not continued to improve as dramatically.

Mrs. Bartell came to understand that the severity of her condition was chemically induced but made worse by her behavioral patterns of denial and avoidance—engaging in palliatives such as the use of ice packs, and continuing to work even with severe pain. Even more fundamentally, she feels she has changed tremendously. She used to be "a workhorse" and tried to please people, exhausting herself in the process and, in her words, she "lost sight of who I was." Her attitude toward her illness was, "This is not going to beat me." Her father had been critically ill and she was taking on all the responsibility for his care. She realized from the healing intensive that it took too much energy to be the stoic person she used to be. Now she finds it easier to ask for help, to say no and rely on other people. She told her brother that she needed help to care for her father and would not do it alone anymore. In her own words, she would "no longer be a doormat for her family and their demands." Her experiences at the clinic have helped her to come to terms with her fear of death, her own and her parents', so that she could be with her father when he passed away. Family members, in a half-joking way, attributed her new self to the corrupting influence of alternative medicine.

She also valued her experience of being "a partner" with her physician, which allowed her to reflect on her life and make appropriate changes. Through her journal (she has completed her seventh) she could share her thought patterns with her holistic physicians and from this they could devise treatment regimes. She has sent videotapes and articles about alternative medicine to her allergist hoping to educate him, but to no avail thus far. She has also experimented with different diets and food regimes although she has found it difficult to sustain her commitment in this respect. In response to Dr. Madrona's somewhat forced departure from the hospital, she wrote a letter to the editor protesting his firing and asked, "How could they take away someone who has done so much good for so many people?" She was quite upset about Madrona's departure.

Jill Downey was involved in a serious car accident in 1996 when she was blindsided by an out of control car. She sustained serious back and neck injuries that resulted in major surgery, including neck fusion. She also sustained serious nerve damage and experiences numbness throughout her back. She suffered chronic sleep deprivation and her injuries resulted in a loss of memory. As a result, her life deteriorated, making it difficult to work in the small business she owned and operated. She was told she would have chronic pain for the rest of her life. A surgical anesthesiologist who administered a series of nerve block injections throughout her back treated her. The treatment did not work and she experienced difficulty walking and pain in her right leg. She then underwent myofacial release (by a physical therapist), and therapy to address the consequences of the original injury (compensations and distortion of posture), which had caused tendinitis and related problems. She also underwent painful treatment to break up scar tissue. While doing her daily exercises recommended by her physical therapist she dislocated her shoulder, causing her to spend four months in rehabilitation and more pain. Every morning she would wake up "and wait for the pain to rock through my body." She continues to see a physical therapist on a regular basis to reduce spasms in her neck and back. The "loss of independence" caused by her injuries and pain was "frustrating and humiliating, and was one of the worst experiences I think I had ever had to deal with."

Her primary doctor (who practiced at the same hospital as the clinic) referred her to the complementary medicine clinic. In all likelihood this referral was a result of Jill's belief that she had suffered as a result of her treatment by conventional medicine—surgical mistakes, the nerve blocks, which resulted in partial paralysis, and physical therapy, which resulted in the shoulder separation, making her bitter and mistrustful since the "healers" who were supposed to help her actually harmed her. She wanted treatment that was "softer." She talked to the administrative director at the clinic for more than two hours in order to determine her therapeutic options and whom she should see for treatment. She wound up seeing one of the more spiritually oriented holistic physicians at the clinic. Perhaps the administrative director recommended this physician because Jill had strong religious and spiritual beliefs and a strong desire to "heal herself" despite the persistent recommendations of her doctors that she had to live with her injuries and that "she would never be the person she was." Her attitude going into the clinic was, "Put me on the fast track to healing. I'll do whatever it takes." In addition she had "a desire to be free from medication" in part as a result of her mother's influence who had not taken a pill for forty-five years. Her mother was also a devout Catholic and this influenced Jill, although Jill's sense of spirituality seems to be more spiritual and less tied to specific religious beliefs.

What she found most helpful was the EMDR treatment she received for the psychological trauma caused by her injuries (including depression). Along with EMDR (an experimental treatment that utilizes rapid eye movement to treat various types of trauma) she was also treated with kinesiology. This technique is based on the principle that past crises and traumas become locked in the form of body memories that are located in various organs or tissues and can be released by this technique. In other words, as she puts it, "emotions have a cellular basis." In part as a result of her treatment, Jill came to believe (at least at the time of her treatment) that energy fields surround the body and that they can be reorganized or altered to achieve a therapeutic effect. Energy is blocked as result of a trauma or injury and this needs to be released. The techniques through which this blocked energy is released ranges from meditation and prayer to massage and manipulating the energy by placing hands a few inches over body. Jill recognized the existence of a "patient culture" at the clinic but "did not partake in it" because "there is only so much pain one can handle," and she was also concerned that this culture could trap someone in a permanent sick role unless it encouraged the patient to "graduate."

Upon reflecting on her treatment, Jill isn't sure whether emotions cause cellular damage or the causal order is the reverse, bodily trauma results in emotional trauma. She is skeptical as well about her physician's spiritually oriented approach that understands disease and bodily injury as vehicles for the expression of higher or deeper and more profound metaphysical and spiritual meanings. In this view her car accident may have been necessary and even intended in order to bring her to a new state of spiritual well-being. She worries that this view would result in patients being blamed for their own illnesses. For Jill, both conventional and alternative medicine have their limitations. At one extreme in alternative medicine there is a kind of spiritual voluntarism where pain can be removed if the person can enter into the right spiritual and psychological state. On the other hand, in conventional medicine the problem for Jill was its overconfidence in its material interventions and when these didn't work counseling resignation and coping with limitations. In her succinct summary, there are the contrasting claims of "you can heal yourself," and, on the other hand, "I will heal you." She was also concerned that medicine "imposes rigid definitions" on the patient and as a result patients see themselves in the rigid categories of the medical system.

Despite her reservations with the approach taken by her holistic physician, Jill believes that her treatment was a "profound experience" that helped her to achieve at least partial independence and freedom from pain. She says, "I'm in process," by which she means in the process of healing, and feels confident this will happen. She continues to work with practitioners at the clinic where she receives both EMDR, energy medicine, and kinesiology. She is back at her old job that is central to her identity and has achieved greater independence.

For both Aime and Jill, it is not likely that either would have ever seen an alternative practitioner if it were not for the complementary medicine clinic's official connection to a hospital. This gave the clinic an imprimatur of legitimacy and scientific standing. In addition, this also made it easier for doctors at the hospital to refer them to the clinic. The setting also allows for collaboration between alternative practitioners so that patients may be treated more holistically. For example, Aime said that during her week-long healing intensive she saw many practitioners during each day, each practitioner with a different modality and all in consultation with one another. Moreover, the setting also allows for conventional and holistic physicians and practitioners to discuss and even debate their respective protocols. This institutional proximity between alternative and conventional medicine may also work to the benefit of conventional medicine in that doctors will be exposed and perhaps may be more willing to accept information and protocols that come out of a different setting. After all, patients at the clinic typically suffer from a range of chronic diseases and have had limited success with conventional doctors. If alternative protocols allow some patients to find relief from symptoms then this information may be of interest to doctors and provide a motive to expand the range of treatments. The fact that complementary medicine clinics are asked to engage in institutional research and keep track of their patients and the efficacy of their interventions makes it possible to provide arguments for extending health care insurance to alternative medical treatments.

The problem with the institutional setting, as stated earlier, is that alternative therapies may be limited in their degrees of experimentation and innovation because of the requirement of constant review by the hospital and the research methodologies that they impose. For example, Dr. Madrona wanted to increase Aime's intravenous dosage of vitamins but was prevented from doing so by the hospital board. More significantly, Dr. Madrona, who was largely responsible for the popularity and innovative programs at the clinic, was forced to leave because of some of his unorthodox techniques, such as the healing intensive and the sweat lodge. The very fact that there is such a highly visible institutional setting makes alternative medicine a target for being labeled "quacks" by groups and organizations that are out to impose their view of what science and proper medicine are. Perhaps, what was discussed earlier as an advantage of institutionalization can also be seen from another perspective as a problem. Patients who could find more innovative and aggressive treatments in the larger submerged networks of alternative health may or may not be willing to utilize this resource because of the existence of an alternative health setting with more legitimacy. For example, both Aime and Jill, despite their largely positive experience at the clinic have had limited contact with the larger alternative health community. They may come to define alternative health as synonymous with the complementary medicine clinic. Aime has become a booster for the clinic, because of their successful treatment of her condition but this has not translated, at this point, into becoming an alternative health activist.

Finally, the very label of the clinic as "complementary" may provide the justification for keeping alternative medicine in its place as if it were something secondary and maybe even peripheral to the core practice of medicine. For example, Jill was only referred to the clinic after the surgery, nerve blocks, and physical therapy failed and, as a result, Jill became angry and blamed her doctors. The hope may have been that the clinic would provide a psychological palliative that would diffuse her anger and forestall possible potential legal action. Clearly, the physical interventions of biomedicine in this view are seen as primary while alternative medicine becomes akin to the work of religion, providing consolation and therapeutic support.

The Clinical Director

We can appreciate the challenges of integrating alternative and conventional medicine from another point of view. Dr. Madrona, a well-known alternative or holistic M.D., was introduced in chapter 3. As the reader may recall, Dr. Madrona wrote about his journey from a career as a conventional physician, trained in one of the leading medical schools, to a growing disenchantment with biomedicine and a rediscovery of his Native American roots. Dr. Madrona is interested in mind-body approaches to healing, some of which are based on traditional Native American healing techniques, and has a strong interest in research. He is pursuing this interest in research through ongoing studies on alternative treatments for autism, asthma, and arthritis, among others. He wound up in Pittsburgh as director of the clinic and later as program director. We interviewed him in the Complementary Medicine Clinic itself as well as the Family Practice Clinic across the street where he spends half of his time.

After agreeing to shift from medical to program director in order to utilize his talents in developing creative treatment regimes, Dr. Madrona developed programs that appropriated elements of traditional approaches to healing. In the "healing intensives" patients entered something akin to the "healing societies" of the Algonquin Indians in which patients would progress together through various stages toward the healing of their illnesses. Encouraging the "waiting room culture" is another means by which patients are encouraged to form relationships of support with one another. Finally, Dr. Madrona on occasion employs "community interventions"—inviting all his diabetes patients to come to the clinic for an afternoon in order to "interact with each other, heal each other and talk to each other. This is something we can learn from traditional healers: Native American, traditional Jewish, shamans." He also recognizes that alternative health regimes require as much or more of a commitment from family members and caregivers as it does from patients, so he often invites his patients to bring family and friends to discuss how they can contribute to the patient's path to healing.

When patients first come to see him he tries to weed out those who are still attached to the model of expertise employed in biomedicine by asking them to research their illness on the internet and to read a number of articles. Those who come back with ideas and questions are the patients he wants to keep. Taken together these approaches seek to radically undermine the professional model of expertise in conventional medicine through treating patients collectively, actively encouraging patients to help one another, and finally through encouraging a relationship of partnership and collaboration between himself and his patients. Dr. Madrona's best guess about why he, in particular, came under attack by prominent physicians at the hospital and by a local "quack buster" group is that as the clinic became more successful and visible, it represented more of a threat. Madrona is also the most visible element in an increasingly visible clinic, having written a semiautobiographical book attacking conventional medicine and giving frequent interviews to newspapers, TV stations, and others.

But perhaps it is Madrona's popularity with the interns and residents that has seemed most threatening to elements of the medical establishment in the hospital. His afternoon rounds in the Family Clinic puts him in contact with residents who consult with him about their patients. He has also been assigned a number of medical students as assistants. We witnessed a number of occasions when he combined conventional medical advice with elements of alternative medicine (nutritional advice for a blood pressure patient, for example). The fact that Madrona is well known and respected among the residents makes his forays into alternative medicine more credible.

> What's funny to me about the whole controversy is that I have this theory, that because I like conventional medicine that that's what makes me controversial. It works really well with the residents. When I'm working with them every day they are more likely to believe me when I tell them about onions and garlic. It hasn't worked that way with the hospital powers that be.

Dr. Madrona's longstanding interest in research has also resulted in friction with elements of the biomedical establishment. He is adamantly opposed to the "religion of double blind trials." While recognizing that these large-scale controlled studies have some value in testing new drugs, he is critical of their exclusive use in evaluating alternative treatment regimes.

> I would argue that the religion of the randomized control trial is probably just that. It isn't the most appropriate research design for

everything and I understand its logic for drug studies. They have large populations and they are looking for side effects and some measure of efficacy and they think they can control by randomizing. It has actually never been shown that you can control variance by randomizing because you just confuse the variance rather than control it. To say that we have randomized so we don't have to worry about confounding variables is naive. When you are randomizing you are not even sure you are randomizing on the right variables.

Dr. Madrona's research on an experimental treatment for autism illustrates, he argues, the limitations of the randomized controlled trial. His research on the use of a nueropeptide—secretin—as a treatment for autism has shown some success but in a randomized trial of twenty patients (performed elsewhere) no therapeutic effect could be demonstrated. The problem with this, according to Madrona, is that little if anything is known about the etiology of autism, so there is no understanding of "what to randomize on." Autism, after all, is a behavioral not a biochemical diagnosis so "what's the logic for randomization?" It may turn out to be the case that there are many subtypes of autism that are amenable to a variety of treatments. Qualitative designs, he argues, also have their place and should receive some funding. For example, we might want to know why some autistic kids improve after receiving secretin. Watching these kids carefully and recording detailed observations on how they have improved might be a good first step in understanding why this treatment works for some children and not others.

Depression is another chronic illness that requires an emphasis on "subtle distinctions," distinctions that are methodologically excluded in the randomized trial.[7]

> Randomized trials look for robust effects applicable to large populations and so miss smaller subgroups. This has probably limited our understanding of depression. So as a physician you probably have no idea which drug to try for depression except which kind of pen you are holding. If you are happening to hold a Prozac pen then you'll prescribe that. In Chinese medicine there's a way of saying that your kind of depression responds better to these herbs whereas your kind of depression responds better to these herbs. There's more discriminating power in Chinese medicine than in allopathic medicine. So I think that institutional factors affect our gaze. We have a Kmart gaze. We look for big categories rather than subtle distinctions.

Madrona attributes this "religion of the randomized trial" to the Anglo-American intellectual culture, which has emphasized empiricism and rationalism, in contrast to the German and continental traditions. In addition, the power of the pharmaceutical companies in America may also be a factor in that the dominant research protocol in bio-medicine is well suited to the large-scale use of pharmaceutical drugs. Ironically, the NIH Office of Alternative Medicine is moving toward the exclusive use of randomized trials for evaluating alternative treatments, making it more difficult for Madrona and others on the clinic staff to do the kind of research they believe will demonstrate the efficacy of alternative medicine.

How does Madrona view the possibility of integration between alternative and conventional medicine? Dr. Madrona is uncomfortable with both the categories of alternative and conventional medicine because he would like to see an emphasis on "medicine that works," or what is now called "evidence-based medicine."[8] This necessitates, in his view, a pragmatic approach that allows for a wide range of treatment modalities as long as it can be demonstrated that the pro-posed treatment is either effective with tolerable side effects or harmless and ineffective. Unfortunately, he argues, much of the treatment offered in conventional medicine is not supported by scien-tific evidence. According to a 1978 report from the Congressional Office of Technology Assessment, only 20 percent of what's done in conventional medicine is supported or suggested by research data. The rest, in Madrona's words, is "tradition and trial and error." According to Goldstein, randomized clinical trials, epidemiological studies, and outcome evaluations conducted by a range of federal agencies have not arrived at conclusions that depart much from this 1978 study.[9] While high-risk procedures such as bone marrow transplants and chemotherapy do not produce demonstrable results (a recent study shows that bone marrow transplants are ineffective), the clinic cannot get approval for an intravenous vitamin treatment that Madrona wants even though at worst the treatment would be ineffective but harmless. His view is that "if you get to do bone marrow transplants, I get to do intravenous vitamins."

The other side of this is Madrona's uneasiness with alternative medicine's "faddishness," which he believes is a result of getting too caught up in specific treatments and approaches and thereby losing sight of what is most valuable about alternative medicine, empowering patients to participate in the healing process through activating their beliefs and through supporting one another. His view of the cancer clinics in Mexico that offer alternative treatments for cancer is that "they simplify and collapse very complex phenomena." The clinics he visited "tend to become focused on a narrow approach in a little bit of a fanatical way." This part of the alternative health landscape (alternative cancer clinics) is the least institutionalized, offering treatments to the terminally ill that are illegal in the United States and operating entirely outside of the medical-industrial complex. Madrona seems to be arguing that their institutional isolation creates the potential for turning their particular approaches to treating cancer into "miracle cures," a kind of alternative health "magic bullet."

The Challenge of Institutionalization

Complementary medicine clinics are only one way in which alternative medicine is establishing closer links to the medical profession and dominant health care system. Alternative health activists across the country are seeking recognition from insurance companies for their protocols, are establishing "integrative" medicine clinics with sympathetic physicians, are pooling their own resources to form alternative HMOs, and in the process may be redefining their collective identity and redrawing old boundaries. But, we have suggested in this chapter, "integration" or institutionalization must be evaluated not solely in terms of the result, the extent to which alternative health groups achieve the official recognition many of them desire, but instead, in terms of what is gained or lost in the process. How institutionalization is achieved may be as important as whether it is achieved.

It's not hard to understand some of the reasons why health insurance companies and hospitals are looking more favorably at alternative medicine. The cost-cutting drive of HMOs fits nicely into alternative medicine's emphasis on low-tech treatments and prevention. It is interesting to note, in this respect, that there is one other complementary medicine clinic in the city, which is financed by Highmark Blue Cross. In addition, hospitals, in a more competitive health care market, may see alternative medicine as a useful "warm and fuzzy" face that could attract a segment of the market and an opportunity to get a piece of government research funding.

On the other hand, the source of opposition to incorporating elements of alternative medicine into the dominant health care system seems to be coming from some segments of the medical profession. For the first time since the establishment of the hegemony of the medical profession in the early twentieth century, many doctors feel threatened by the spread of the corporate model of organization into medicine. The fear that their professional autonomy and earnings might be seriously jeopardized may result in a heightened sensitivity to the threat from alternative medicine.[10] Here, the threat is not so much to professional autonomy but to scientific legitimacy. Physicians who are organizing against the complementary medicine clinic argue that there is no solid scientific evidence to support the clinic's approaches. This critique, as discussed earlier, is somewhat disingenuous considering the fact that much evidence already exists of the efficacy of mind-body approaches and there are legitimate questions about the appropriate scientific model to use in doing clinical research. Nevertheless, this critique is an effective strategy for conservative forces within the medical profession to fight off a weaker adversary.[11] It is interesting, in this respect, that the support for the clinic comes from a number of prominent members of the board as well as a core of enthusiastic patients. As mentioned earlier, few conventional physicians are willing to work with the clinic staff and some physicians are actively working to shut the clinic down.

The practitioners and directors of the complementary medicine clinic are keenly aware that their continued existence is precarious. Like any bureaucracy the hospital must evaluate the success of each subdivision or department. The problem, though, is that the hospital's standards of efficacy and the clinic's are not compatible. Processing patients through the clinic would require shortening the time patients spend with holistic physicians and practitioners, so it is not likely the clinic can pay its own way without sacrificing its mission. Demonstrating the effectiveness of its treatments through the use of double blind randomized studies also runs counter to the holistic emphasis in alternative medicine—the synergy of patient empowerment, individualized treatment regimes, and multiple modalities.

Ironically, in alternative health faith that alternative medicine is the wave of the future is nearly universal. Much of this faith is grounded in a naive view that the truth will inevitably triumph and that change occurs in a simple way—from lifeworld to institutions. In other words, as people change the way they think about health and illness, institutions will inevitably follow. But there is another possibility. Only those elements of alternative medicine that are consistent with the health care institution's commodified, bureaucratic, and "scientific" form will be incorporated.

A possible scenario is that more and more people will buy herbs, minerals, and vitamins, and pharmaceutical companies will find a way to profit from this. Complementary medicine clinics, if they are to continue, will focus on profit-making services, such as acupuncture, massage, and prescribing herbs and vitamins. Alternative health promoters will make more money on books, courses, and services. HMOs will find ways to incorporate elements of alternative medicine that they believe will reduce health care costs. Alternative health practitioners in their continuing efforts to enhance their credentials and status will adopt the model of expertise modeled after the medical system whereby the doctor is the expert and monopolizes medical information. And finally, alternative modalities that are the least holistic are likely to be the only ones to survive the rigors of biomedical research. Branches of alternative medicine that claim a fundamental incompatibility with conventional medicine will be marginalized. In other words, alternative health will become absorbed into market relations and structures of bureaucratic power.[12]

The danger here is that alternative health activists will get caught up in this process of institutionalization and as a result lose their movement character as a kind of anarchic flow of information, remedies, and modalities that are potentially innovative, pathbreaking, and at times dangerous. In any social movement, as we have mentioned, there is a dialectic between the more institutionalized segments and its "submerged networks." The more the institutionalized segments dominate, the greater the danger of the drying up of creativity and innovation that are rooted in the flows of interaction in the lifeworld. An excess of creativity may result from the other type of imbalance, when noninstitutionalized segments dominate. Here a wide range of approaches to health and illness may blossom but the achievement of an ongoing collaboration between practitioners and patients as well as a systematic learning process is problematic. The opportunities for hucksterism (miracle cures), scams, and wild conspiratorial theories may blossom under these conditions.

In alternative health there is a less than full appreciation of the challenge of translating the gains made on the micro level to the institutional level. As a result the full benefit of retaining the tension between the submerged, anarchic networks and institutionalization is underappreciated. If the links connecting the two levels of power within the alternative health movement are severed it will lose what makes it "alternative"—an effort to reconnect health and illness to the lifeworlds of patients.

While we have argued that alternative health must remain a dual movement, the power of the movement in the final analysis rests upon the fact that it is embedded in the practices of the lifeworld. It is that level that provides spaces for discovery and innovation, and models of interaction that are nonbureaucratic and noncommodified, in other words, the basis for a value shift. This value shift creates the potential for translation into institutional and policy changes. As Habermas puts it, it is cultural innovation at the level of the lifeworld that provides the pathway for larger social change.

We might apply this thesis with respect to health and illness in the following way. As people cope with problems in their lives such as chronic illness, they discover and utilize new practices that suggest new horizons of value and meaning, the roots of which we have tried to specify through our discussion of the auratic character of the products and practices of alternative health. In this way illness becomes reembedded in new contexts, which challenge mechanistic models of the body, and our instrumental relationship to nature. The dual movement character of alternative health may be suggestive of a model for any social movement. If the links between the institutional character of the movement and its lifeworld practices are severed a social movement risks becoming co-opted, a mere embroidery on the status quo. The other danger is that meanings and redefinitions of the self may change without any institutional forming effect and as a result people become alienated from the world around them. We try to clarify the larger stakes involved in the concluding chapter.

Conclusion

Alternative Health and Colonization

We argue in this book that alternative health should not be conceived narrowly as an alternative medical practice, but instead that it is more fruitful to analyze it as a social movement. It is a social movement because it plays an important role in a value shift emerging within the textures of everyday life and provides energies for new associations that have a wider potential for social change. The products and practices of alternative health suggest a noninstrumental relation to the world. We've tried to capture this noninstrumental relation through Benjamin's conception of the aura and the way this releases images of reconciliation of nature within the lifeworld. We use the word *suggest* because this valorization of the natural is not fundamentally discursive but originates in flashes that intimate a sense of finding one's home and a feeling of safety in a manufactured world moving in the opposite direction.

We have also shown that in alternative health patients practice regimes that have a family resemblance to what Foucault has called "technologies of the self." The mastery of the self through these regimes attempts to order lives in terms of the perfection of nature that is suggested through a variety of auratic experiences. Furthermore, technologies of the self open people to wider social and political involvements. In other words, through cultural experimentation on the

183

level of the lifeworld, patients are more likely to become active in other movement networks and even higher levels of formal organization. We have begun our analysis with the lifeworld because it is here, we believe, that alternative health makes its fundamental contribution to social change. We have shown that on the level of everyday practices alternative health participants, in both networks, share a critique of the health care system and other elements of modern societies.

We have demonstrated that the movement from emergent horizons of meaning to social action can be more fully understood in the context of Habermas's theory of colonization. Alternative health is bound up with the "colonization of the lifeworld" both as resistance and as a form of accommodation. People enter into the world of alternative health not because of ideology but typically because of a range of chronic illnesses, which are not being satisfactorily treated by conventional medicine. In other words, the travails of the body is the motor that leads to involvement in alternative health. Once patients shift their medical environment, resistance to colonization becomes a possibility.

According the Habermas, colonization produces two pathological consequences. First, there is a loss of autonomy as patients become subject to control and direction by bureaucratic systems and the market. In personal terms, the expert monopolizes medical knowledge and health care practices. Secondly, there is a loss of meaning. Disease is treated mechanically and divested of larger moral significance. The body becomes a mechanism rearranged through the intervention of drugs and surgery. Alternative health responds to colonization by partially resisting the loss of meaning. At the most basic level disease is reenchanted. Disease is understood as a consequence of a fall from the inherent harmony and balance in nature. In the Christian network we studied this perfect order is grounded in biblical principles, while in the holistic network the natural is supported through a variety of invented traditions. Disease poses questions for the totality of one's life and how it's lived rather than being an arbitrary result of external forces that overtake the body. In other words, in alternative health disease teaches us something about life and its fundamental character.

What weakens this resistance, at the most basic level, is that the evocation of nature comes by the way of a variety of fragmented traditions that a person chooses from. People are not in any one emphatic tradition that evokes the natural world without qualification. Instead, people choose among the ruins of traditions that only imply or suggest a different relation between society and the natural world.

What also weakens this experience of enchantment and its discursive expressions is the way alternative health is increasingly bound up with the market and entrepreneurial activity. When herbs, vitamins, and minerals are marketed and sold like any drug or commodity their unique and auratic character is drained away. Herbs, for instance, can become magic bullets working as mechanically as drugs and merchandised as such. Insofar as alternative health becomes a niche market, it becomes just another business in competition with the pharmaceutical industry. At this level, herbs do not provide means of transforming or reordering one's life. They are simply instances of the latest health fad.

Alternative health also has a complex relation to the question of autonomy and social transformation. Its cultivation of technologies of the self helps to contest the monopoly of health care by experts. This compels a challenge to the authority of the doctor and the accompanying "sick role." Technologies of the self involve a learning process where people actively pursue knowledge about health and disease and a mastery of health practices. Further, this self-mastery provides an opening into wider forms of activism that emerges out of their holistic understanding of chronic disease. Properly conceived, holism challenges the reductionism of biomedicine and therefore the efficacy and legitimacy of medical authority. To the extent to which holism relates the totality of factors that shape the health and well-being of the body it becomes intrinsically politicizing. Chronic disease can be understood as the way the body registers the pathologies of the modern world, as a passive template to which the person succumbs. Technologies of the self respond to this politicized notion of disease through daily practices of resistance. In contrast, the sick role has no socially transforming possibility.

What is weak about alternative health's resistance to colonization in this context is the desire of many in the movement to become an institutionally sanctioned force and a subordinate aspect of the biomedical system. Alternative medicine becomes biomedicine's warm and fuzzy face. Insofar as practitioners desire credentials and seek professional recognition the dual movement character of the movement is threatened. As alternative health becomes professionalized, practitioners too may pursue a monopoly of expertise and dry out the roots of the movement. Finally, we have argued that alternative health is only partially holistic and tends to depart from its potential. There are varieties of alternative medicine that give causal priority to spiritual and psychological factors as unilateral sources of diseases, thereby neglecting social, environmental, and political factors. Throughout alternative health this larger dimension is neglected, which weakens its capacity to challenge the larger social order. In summary, while the processes of commodification and professionalization weaken alternative health's capacity to resist colonization, alternative health cannot be reduced to these processes.

Alternative Health; Premodern, Modern, or Postmodern?

The fact that large numbers of people are moving toward alternative health should not be understood only in terms of questions about the efficacy of biomedicine but instead seen in terms of wider cultural shifts. It may be useful in this respect to examine alternative health in light of the dominant social trend, "postmodernism." At the core of the postmodern project is its rejection of modernism and its grand narratives of progress. In other words, postmodernism begins with the critique of the view that history moves in a unified upward direction from barbarism to enlightenment, from poverty to wealth, from slavery to freedom, and from superstition and magic to truth through science and its various avatars such as biomedicine. Alternative health partially shares this postmodernist critique. The failure of biomedicine to give meaning to as well as to effectively treat a wide range of chronic illnesses opens up a space for sympathy with postmodernism. Alternative health resists the Cartesian world view of biomedicine, which separates mind and body and its advocacy of the mechanical intervention into nature that strives to manufacture health. In alternative health knowledge is context bound, resistant to universalizing rules applicable to all. The dream in biomedicine is to discover a biological mechanism responsible for each disease and to eventually understand disease on the molecular level. The goal is to isolate the biological mechanism responsible for a disease and the gene that triggers this mechanism. Eventually the goal is to manipulate the gene and cure the disease. The emphasis is on understanding and treating specific diseases (rather than individual sickness) so that all individuals can be treated, more or less, the same way. But in alternative medicine, and even among some primary care physicians within biomedicine, "disease" cannot exist a part from the total ecology of the person. Such a view resists the tendency toward universalization since every patient must be treated differently. The clinical sensitivity to the specific ecology of the patient is subordinated to the anonymous universalizing approach of biomedicine. This condition is arguably rooted in institutional pressures—the specialization of medical expertise, the links between medicine and the pharmaceutical industry and dominant models of scientific research. Alternative health does not reject evidence-based practices but shifts its definition in an individualizing direction. What constitutes evidence becomes the issue.

Within biomedicine the evidentiary standard is the isolation of the underlying mechanism that brings about a cure or the relief of symptoms. On the other hand, in much of alternative medicine, evidence consists of whether or not the person experiences health and well-being through a range of integrated treatments designed to affect the specific ecology of the person. This commitment to an ecological view of the person bears a family resemblance to tendencies in postmodernism with respect to their pragmatic orientation toward truth.[1] In other words, there are certain affinities between alternative health and the pragmatic approach, which argues that the question to ask in not whether it is true but whether it works.

However, a more finely grained analysis shows some differences between postmodernism and alternative health. Alternative health's commitment to an ecological rather than reductionist view of the patient has an essentialist component that to some degree takes it out of the modern world. This involves a kind of naiveté with respect to the "natural" and traditional worlds, which are celebrated. This naiveté puts them to some degree in tension with the pragmatic orientation of their health practices. This tension can be understood in the following way. In terms of their practices alternative health is for the most part pragmatic, although there are groups that have a dogmatic commitment to a particular set of protocols such as macrobiotics. But, for the most part, when it comes to the reflective explanation and justification of these practices the tendency is to be essentialist—their practices have to conform to the preexisting harmony in nature. In other words, the treatment of illness involves a cocktail of natural remedies that are tailored through trial and error to the specific ecology of the person. On another level, when it comes to the justification of these practices simpliciter, the metaphysical and aesthetic language of balance and harmony is invoked. What ties these two levels together, the essentialist notion of nature as a symmetrical order and the pragmatism of their approach to health, is that the health regimes recommended consist of remedies that are not humanly created or manufactured.

Postmodernism as well addresses questions of nature and tradition but only ironically and in the form of a semantic play of signifiers. But in alternative health the attainment of a more natural state through the auratic connection with the past is a fundamental drive that sweeps throughout the movement. This orientation toward the natural allows alternative health to have a different relationship to the modern world than postmodernism. Postmodernism's rejection of utopianism[2] means that any notion of the natural as a source of collective action or identity is erased in order to guard against the dangers of the grand narratives of progress and other illusions. In contrast, alternative health's celebration of the natural through romanticized images of nature gives it a weak utopian character around which groups can form.

In brief, alternative health appears to have some resemblance to postmodern conceptions of truth at the level of its practices but its valorization of nature gives it the appearance of being premodern. We could say, therefore, that alternative health floats between these two poles. The premodern character of alternative health consists of its celebration of traditions and use of ritualized health care practices. Alternative health's commitment to the values of modernity takes the form of its resistance to medical authority, and its commitment to self-care and autonomy. When a movement floats uneasily between established symbolic markers, none of which can account for and fully explain its practice, this perhaps suggests that it is the source of a new constellation of values and orientations whose character depends on the way it is filtered and taken up by higher levels of social organization.

From Lifeworld to Politics

According to the pragmatist tradition, people are able to make cognitive gains when their preconceived plans of action can no longer be carried out because of unexpected obstacles that emerge in their lives.[3] When action becomes interrupted people become aware of the merely subjective character of their beliefs because these beliefs no longer allow them to act effectively in the world, to go on without problems. In this way, people encounter themselves as interpreters of their world. We'd like to take this insight and apply it to illness and the body. Illness is perhaps the most fundamental way in which everyday life is interrupted for actors. The body is no longer an instrument for our purposes but is an "other" that resists us.[4] These interruptions present opportunities for a person to reweave the fabric of her life and create new configurations of meaning. When this interruption can no longer be relieved through traditionally sanctioned forms of medical intervention (as is the case with most chronic illnesses), it may lead, and empirically it increasingly does lead, to alternative health care strategies. This engagement with alternative health is not simply a competing medical practice. Because of alternative health's auratic qualities it stimulates people to reembed illness and by extension the self in a new framework of meaning. The experiential roots of this framework, as we have argued, are the flashes of reconciliation that are suggested by the auras that surround alternative health products and practices. These auratic experiences enable people to become more open to discursive arguments that attempt to rethink fundamentally a different relation between society, institutions, and the natural world.

These discourses circulate within the three levels of power that Offe identifies. In the microsphere of everyday life, alternative health makes its contribution through the circulation of images of reconciliation with the natural world. At the second level, the level of competing movements and interest groups, alternative health as a social movement advocates nonindustrial farming, resistance to drug-based therapies, the simplification of everyday life, a reorientation of life away from narrowly instrumental definitions of success, and a legally supported pluralistic health care system. This advocacy partially resists commodification and more completely attacks the bureaucratization of health care.

What remains to be discussed is Offe's third level, in which politicians communicate with experts on public policy. Here the relation between images that float in the microsphere of everyday life and the technical analyses of experts seems the most stretched but nevertheless it is not severed. Value shifts, and their experiential roots within everyday life, provide the context within which experts do their work and draw their support. The experiential openness of people to arguments and policies that are offered on this third level depends on value shifts within the microsphere of everyday life. We have shown in a concrete way a solution to the problem that Habermas poses concerning the way theoretical gains of expert cultures can be released into everyday life and transform it in a rational direction. We've demonstrated this through our analysis of the compromised nature of expertise in alternative health because alternative health experts live off the practices and traditions in the lifeworld. Alternative health experts, as we have argued, modify but do not break away from the everyday competencies of people that are given to them through tradition. Also, in contrast to Habermas, who emphasizes enlightenment in one direction from experts to everyday actors, we emphasize the way in which the lifeworld and the experiences of actors provide the resources that experts draw upon to do their work.[5] Both the lifeworld and the expert culture of alternative health mutually interact to provide the basis for a value shift.

This reciprocal interaction provides a model to understand value shifts that are more global than health and disease. To illustrate, one significant way in which the value shift on the level of everyday life becomes condensed into discourses is through the language of "sustainable development." Modern economics, along with biomedicine, is rooted in the world view of Cartesianism. Schumpeter calls this Cartesian influence on classical economics its preanalytic vision.[6] This vision assumes a certain implicit relationship between people and the natural world. People are conceptualized as independent from the constraints of the natural world. This means that there are no natural limits to economic growth because of the infinite capacity of human knowledge and creativity, which can completely replace the constraints of nature. Classical economics can only deal with nature as an externality and therefore secondary to the workings of their central models.

A sustainable system of economics, in contrast, would expand this preanalytic vision to include natural capital and the way it puts limits on development. This in turn would lead us to new definitions of economic growth which are not only sustainable but have some clear relationship to human happiness and well-being.[7] These technical arguments by experts in favor of sustainability imply fundamental changes in everyday life that could only be accomplished if people were already open to them to some degree by virtue of their experiences in the lifeworld. Changes in everyday life among participants in alternative health allow a partial receptivity to these views. The gap can only be closed through work on the level of networks and social movements.

How does this value shift, more particularly, shape the understanding of illness as well as the treatment of disease and funding for research in the health care system? This value shift, as we have noted, revolves around an ecological or "holistic" conception of illness and health. In this view, the healthy or ill person is part of a larger web of dependencies and connections. These dependencies include the food we eat, the air we breathe, the work we do, our relationships, the way we spend our free time, the way we move around in the world, among other things. All these considerations ultimately are justified as being in accord with some natural state of balance and harmony with the physical world. The nature in us must be in balance with the nature outside us. Again, the natural confronts us as a pivotal consideration but now we want to examine its policy implications.

The way this evocation of the natural at the level of the lifeworld works its way into higher levels of social movements and policy making is fraught with tension and contradictions that lead to a range of conflicting possibilities. To be in accord with nature can be conceptualized as how the elements that make up the totality of our lives fit together. To work too hard, spend too much, be under too under stress, and eat the wrong kinds of food can be thought of as an expression of an unbalanced or unnatural way of life. In this sense the evocation of the natural and its discursive expressions can lead to receptivity to the connection between disease and what has been called "the total social process." The potential here is for the understanding of illness to connect to a critique of society, its goals, and its institutional structure. This sensibility has a potential that has only been partially taken up at the level of public policy. We already see some alternative protocols for heart disease that include eating natural foods and relaxation techniques being funded by major insurance companies, and HMOs.[8] The government, through the NIH Center for Complementary and Alternative Medicine allocates a modest but growing amount of money for research into alternative health.[9] Corporations for a long time have developed for their white-collar employees "wellness programs" and exercise centers.[10] But the potential is far richer than these limited efforts. We can envision a transformation of the biomedical paradigm in which disease is conceptualized in a richer and more multidimensional manner and research not narrowly constrained by a scientistic closure on the origins and nature of disease. Doctors would then become more pragmatic in their orientations and not limited to drug and surgical interventions.

At the same time, the evocation of the natural influences public policy in other directions. While the natural and its discursive expressions can provide momentum for institutional change, it also can block off an understanding of disease as it relates to wider situational factors. Too often the self descriptions of patients and alternative health activists are drawn from the language of possessive individualism. This is not surprising in a culture that valorizes the power of the individual. In this view nature is a source of guidance for individuals in constructing their lifestyles. It is the responsibility of the person to choose the appropriate natural path and this can always be done independently of institutions and their direction. The natural here creates a kind of existential hubris. This can lead to an insidious remoralization of illness, which leads to self-blame and overconfidence in diagnosis and cure. Susan Sontag has warned of the danger of giving disease an overly metaphorical meaning and its consequent overburdening of the person with guilt and self-blame.[11]

Which of these two potential directions are actualized cannot be derived from the concept of the natural itself but from the way it is taken up by social movements and given particular interpretive understanding. The ability to connect disease to wider social processes, to develop a "diagnoses for our times," is far more difficult to achieve than the pursuit of health as an individual project. To the extent to which alternative health remains on the level of the individual and his or her efforts to become healthy through spiritual, psychological, and lifestyle changes it becomes another element in popular or mass culture. The discourse of "positive thinking," spiritual transformation, and the fitness movement are well integrated in the culture of late capitalist society. There is little potential for social transformation at this level. But an analysis at this level does not capture what is significant about alternative health. As we have argued, the transformation of the self in alternative health creates an opening for wider political involvements as well as a critique of social institutions.

Alternative Health, Social Movements, and Social Capital

Robert Putnam has persuasively documented the decline of social capital in America over the past thirty to forty years. By social capital he refers to the networks of trust and obligation that range from informal visiting, bridge games, bowling leagues, voluntary associations, philanthropy, membership in professional associations, and more explicitly political activities like voting, membership in political parties, and the larger sphere of civic participation. One example illustrates this process. As a percentage of their income, Americans donate less to charities than they did in the 1940s. Moreover, Americans also volunteer less as well. In 1975–76, 40 percent of American adults reported that they worked on some community project over the previous year and in the late nineties that percentage fell to thirty-three percent. Organizations such as the Parent-Teacher Association have also dramatically declined over the past few decades.[12]

It would appear that the rise of new social movements since the 1960s contradicts this thesis. But Putnam argues that most membership in these movements (like the environmental movement) amounts to a yearly donation with little active involvement in the organization itself. The exception to this is the rise of the Christian Right, where the membership is highly active in a wide range of areas.[13] Another exception is the self-help or "small group" movement, recovery groups such as Alcoholics Anonymous and the like.[14] Alternative health as a social movement has a complex relationship to these larger trends that Putnam identifies.

We have argued that participation in alternative health care networks is a form of social capital because it engages people in ongoing activities that are based on mutual assistance, sharing of knowledge, and the development of skilled practices. In this sense alternative health is similar to the Christian Right and self-help or support groups that resist the larger trend of declining social capital. It is significant that alternative health is part of this larger resistance to "bowling alone." What all three—self help, the Christian Right and alternative health—have in common is that for all of them there is a reciprocal interaction between social networks and self-transformation. But there are some important differences. Compared to self-help or support groups, alternative health is not as isolated from wider community associations and involvements. In fact, we have suggested that alternative health connects activists to other movements and networks. In contrast, the evidence is that self-help and support group involvement is not linked to forms of civic participation such as volunteering, voting, or joining social movements. In fact, self-help or support groups are often isolated from the larger community and focused on the individual quests of members.

The relationship between alternative health and the rise of the Christian Right is somewhat more complex. Here we can make use of Habermas's distinction between offensive and defensive new social movements. As discussed earlier, defensive new social movements involve protecting an endangered way of life, however conceived, from the encroachments of bureaucratic and market forces. Offensive new social movements, on the other hand, involve efforts to construct new forms of life. These new forms of life attempt to embody rational potentials that have been unleashed with the emergence of modern society. Put simply, a rational lifeworld involves the increasingly critical and reflective appropriation of knowledge, morality, and personal identity. As a result of the rationalization of the lifeworld, tradition loses its authoritative and emphatic ability to organize human life. Of course, when these new forms of life, such as feminist health collectives, are threatened by pro-family conservatives or by system imperatives in the form of bureaucratic and market forces, they attempt to defend their newly created spaces.

The newly politicized evangelical subculture can be understood as a biblically grounded defense of a traditional way of life—a defense against the welfare state and its encroachments upon the autonomy of families, and the rampant commercialism of a sexually charged and violent mass culture. Alternative health, which includes evangelical groups, has a more contradictory relationship to bureaucratization and commodification. The Christian network we've studied can be understood as a defensive reaction to the system in the name of an invented tradition based on biblical sources. Its commitment to natural remedies is legitimated through religious text. Yet, their involvement in alternative health networks exercises pressure toward rationalization. Through the use of diverse alternative health modalities grounded frequently in non-Western traditions (despite the warnings of some, this is inescapable), people are opened to influences from other metaphysical traditions. As a result, the purity of the tradition becomes "polluted." In addition, Christian alternative health activists come into contact, at their own meetings, at the co-op, and other places, with the carriers of these unwanted traditions and so become pressured to develop a more playful and relativized view of the sources of their health and well-being. The evangelical subculture, in contrast, is more homogenous and isolated, creating an alternative world for participants so that their assumptions are rarely questioned. Through technologies of the self and its antibureaucratic impulse, patients and activists enter into spaces of autonomy that center them squarely in the modern world. Because the basis for self-care in alternative health is pulled from such diverse sources, which the person must creatively appropriate, the person enters a kind of nondogmatic space. In summary, the social capital created through alternative health networks is what Putnam calls "bridging social capital" in contrast to the "bonding social capital" of the larger evangelical Christian subculture.[15] To the extent to which support groups build social capital at all, the evidence is that it is of the "bonding" type. Alternative health is also important because it roots this "bridging" social capital in the persistent travails of the body afflicted with chronic illness.

The Future of Medicine

The growing commitment of people to alternative health care protocols and modalities opens a space for the wider consideration of the sources and treatment of illness. Alternative health, we have argued, distances patients from biomedicine's definition of disease and its cure. That definition relentlessly cuts off illness from an understanding of the "total social process." In the biomedical view all illness involves an interaction between genes and pathogens. What is excluded here is not only everything about the person that cannot be reduced to a biological mechanism but also wider historical, social, and environmental factors. In the biomedical paradigm these wider factors are bracketed so that the reductionist impulse of science to discover underlying biological causes can proceed.

One example may illustrate how we can contextualize disease in a way that challenges the biomedical model. Recent studies have shown that diabetes is one of the fastest growing chronic diseases. Its growth cannot be adequately understood in terms of pathogens or underlying biological mechanism. In the most immediate sense we can understand the "diabetes epidemic" as related to lifestyle issues concerning the amount and type of food one consumes. For instance, type two diabetes is closely connected to the increase of obesity in the population. But even here we can go farther. The increase of "junk food" and its aggressive marketing, and the widespread use of sugar in all foods connects this disease with institutional forces. But we also need to examine class factors as well and how they intersect with these other choices and pressures.[16] In fact, one could make the argument that in all chronic diseases an adequate understanding requires examining how class position shapes the susceptibility of people to illness. It is well known that dietary patterns vary by social class and poorer people are not likely to consume as healthy a diet as more privileged groups. Also, we cannot separate the eating patterns of the working class and poor from the stresses resulting from their condition of powerlessness, in areas ranging from work to school to everyday life. It is now well known that long-term stress can spark the onset of many chronic diseases when combined with more immediate triggers. There are also class-specific forms of stress. According to Lewin, stress in more privileged groups tends to spike and then level off and go downward. Among the working class and poor, stress, when triggered by events, tends to remain high because the conditions that produce it remain present.[17] At a more global level, broad social and political changes produced by commitments to a certain notion of development lead to a food production system that is increasingly harmful.

Cardiovascular disease can also be understood in this larger framework. The idea that heart disease is related to lifestyle and nutrition is almost a truism, but not long ago it was contested.

Contextualizing heart disease in terms of lifestyle is just a beginning. As with diabetes, class factors are central in understanding susceptibility to heart disease. In fact, class position is a better predictor of heart disease than an individual's cholesterol level.[18] What this means is that heart disease is closely related to the inequality of wealth and power that exists in the larger society. In fact, as discussed earlier, recent research shows that social hierarchy of any form is closely correlated with an overall decline in health. The decline in social capital combined with the increasing hours of work that result from a certain conception of economic development leads to lives that are increasingly busy and stressful.

The contextualizing of illness, a perspective consistent with what others have called "social medicine," contests the jurisdiction of biomedicine by politicizing disease.[19] Only in this way can we escape the notion, common in biomedicine and alternative medicine, that illness is either a choice or a result of known or unknown biological processes. If disease is precisely multifactoral then the decreasing success of biomedicine in treating chronic disease can be understood as a consequence of its methodological blindness. Alternative medicine's holistic perspective moves it partially toward the contextualization of disease, but, as discussed earlier, it remains partially trapped in an individualistic model. In this model the source of disease may be multifactoral but the solution is always up to the individual. In this way alternative health's holism is not holistic enough. Despite this limitation, the promise of alternative health is not wholly contained by its dominant practices and understandings of itself. As patients begin to break out of the biomedical model and practice self-care, make connections with other healing traditions, and develop relationships with other movements, people become more available for a more complete and contextualized understanding of disease and its treatment.

What is the future of alternative health in relation to the health care system and its understanding of illness? We postulate, in a preliminary way, a number of ways in which alternative health can be taken up into the practice of health and illness in modern societies. One possibility is that the promise of genetic engineering made possible by the completion of the Genome project will deepen the assumptions of biomedicine and make it more intransigent toward alternative modalities. Funding will drive this process by continuing to de-emphasize clinical experience in favor of high-tech interventions such as organ transplants, robotic surgery, and designer drugs that promise to lengthen the lifespan or even eliminate death.[20] Alternative health will be an embroidery to this core project. Its task will be to treat minor health problems that are not worth the attention of the medical establishment. Alternative medicine will also be given the task of offering spiritual consolation when high-tech medicine fails. This form of "medical pluralism" is compatible with the dominance of biomedicine and we can envision it in a market-based system or a national health system such as Canada's or Great Britain's. The degree of toleration of alternative practitioners would vary widely but at the core of such a system (which exists today in the United States and much of western Europe) is the existence of alternative health at the margins of a health care system dominated by biomedicine. Pressures to employ alternative therapies would come from a continued fiscal crisis in the health care system, and alternative therapies would be seen as cost effective when they do not interfere with the core activities of biomedicine.

Another possible model is a medical system where alternative health plays an important but subordinate role insofar as it can be integrated with biomedicine. Here biomedicine would remain essentially unchallenged but would be supplemented by the use of natural remedies and other alternative therapies. For instance, the treatment of cancer would still involve radiation, surgery, and chemotherapy but would also include utilization of natural supplements that have powerful immune boosting properties, such as shark cartilage and MGM-3, a product derived from medicinal mushrooms. This would affect the training of doctors who would receive some training in nutrition, botanical medicine, homeopathy, energy medicine, and bodywork modalities. Conventional doctors would be more likely in this model to consult with alternative practitioners to develop healing strategies. In fact, doctors may supplement their medical education with degrees in various branches of alternative medicine. In such a model, biomedicine would remain dominant, and doctors would be the final arbiters in deciding what alternative therapies would be recommended, a decision that would be based in large part on subjecting alternative therapies to double blind randomized trials.

A third model is one in which alternative and biomedicine compete on an equal basis as parallel health systems. Patients would be able to choose which service best fits their needs. Such a system is compatible with a national system of health care provision as long as the state no longer provides biomedicine with a legal monopoly. It is probably less compatible with a market-based system modeled after the American model. Large groups of working people and poor people without employer-based health insurance would be denied medical services of any kind and natural remedies are not profitable compared to pharmaceuticals and the manufacture of sophisticated medical technology. Of course, as Cant and Sharma point out, the state would have a role in regulation, ensuring that public expenditures are not wasted and consumers are protected.[21] But, this role as watchdog would not involve demands that all alternative therapies be subjected to clinical trials modeled after the testing of pharmaceuticals. Other methods of scientific testing of alternative health therapies would be devised. This model would be one of true pluralism, in contrast to what exists today.

In the final model, alternative and conventional medicine would disappear into a new paradigm. In this paradigm, whose features we have tried to outline with our notion of contextualizing disease, we would see health and illness in relationship to the total social process. In this model, concerns not addressed within the present health care system or by alternative medicine would become central. These concerns are already being introduced by a variety of social movements such as the environmental justice movement,[22] which seeks to address issues of the impact of pollution and the storing and burning of toxic waste material on the working class, poor, and minorities. The emphasis in social medicine on the connection between broader social inequalities and health would also be incorporated as would be the environmental movement's focus on the relationship between economic development and the ecosystem. For all three of these movements—ecology, environmental justice, and social medicine—the pursuit of health cannot be limited to the reductionist project of biomedicine. Instead, health is indissolubly part of the reconstruction of society as a whole.

Alternative health's part in this new paradigm will be to focus our attention on redefining what health care is, asking the question of what is health and illness. Health and illness will be reintegrated into more fundamental questions about the totality of a person's life and the factors that shape it. The point here is not to make biomedicine more accessible but to transform the understanding of health and illness. Alternative health also suggests through its valorization of the natural that something is wrong with the direction of modern society and its conception of progress. In contrast to the social justice emphasis in social medicine and the environmental justice movement, alternative health's implicit critique of progress connects the question of the direction of society and its bearing upon health to the notion of happiness.

As we mentioned earlier, Walter Benjamin understood happiness to involve a renewal of the semantic potentials that are embedded in tradition, passed along through the generations. This gives us a kind of world in which we are situated but which is not at our disposal to use instrumentally. Alternative health suggests these worlds and therefore "rubs history against the grain." Through the appropriation of other healing traditions and the forms of life embedded in them, suggestions of different relations of people to one another, noncommodified understandings of time and space, and forms of wisdom concerning the right ways to live are preserved. Of course these forms of life are not simply preserved without qualification but are rewoven in response to new challenges. The other movements, such as social medicine and environmental justice, provide the conditions for a good life but not its substance. These movements try to equalize the chances for illness by eliminating their class and race specific character. But they do not allow people to cope with the immediate experience of their illness or provide paths to overcome the suffering connected to it. Instead, to be truly healthy is inseparable from renewing the forms of life embedded in the past, however partially. This renewal of the past provides a sense of continuity that situates people within larger contexts. In this way people are not isolated in coming to terms with illness and can find meaning in it.

Another contribution of alternative health to this new paradigm is its commitment to the reskilling of the person and the way it serves to mediate the relation between experts and everyday life. It therefore extends the question of health and illness to a broader project of democratizing health care, which becomes the care of the self. The patient becomes a partner with practitioners who are no longer the monopolized providers of health. As people expand their practices in self-care, they provide the basis for expanding their understanding of the sources of illness. If a person is actively caring for his own illness and inevitably runs up against limits, such as the nature of his work or the lack of availability of healthy foods, or allergies caused by air pollution, he becomes open to a broader understanding of why he is not well and what it would take to become better. This expanded awareness is not blocked by institutional interests. We could say that the demonopolization of health care by experts provides an opportunity for understanding the social and political sources of illness. This in turn would transform and enrich health care practices.

The implementation of this new paradigm may well require a new movement that will draw upon elements of ecology, social medicine, environmental justice, alternative health, and others in developing a viable alternative to biomedicine without sacrificing biomedicine's contributions. If, as many argue, biomedicine is intimately linked to the rise of corporate capitalism, then this new paradigm will require far-reaching changes in society beyond the sphere of health care. So any new movement that will fuse demands for a more just health care system, as well as a more democratic and meaningful one, can succeed only as part of larger social change efforts.

In short, alternative health has a unique role to play in this emerging paradigm. Yet it cannot fulfill its own possibilities by itself whether in a model where it is subordinate, equal, or integrated with biomedicine. It is blind to the question of institutional power and how this shapes the provision of health care. Too often trapped by the market model of health, it doesn't see how its own interests can be better served in a different system of health care provision. Often, natural remedies and products are unavailable because they have no commercial value, yet there's little emphasis in alternative health on the role of the market in foreclosing access to them. Though it's hard to specify all the details of this new paradigm, alternative health's emphasis on autonomy and a renegotiated relationship to nature will be indispensable.

Notes

Introduction

1. The high percentage of women in our sample is consistent with research that shows a high percentage of women among alternative health practitioners and activists. See Sarah Cant and Ursula Sharma, *A New Medical Pluralism? Alternative Medicine, Doctors, and the State* (New York: UCL Press, 2001), 75–7. This issue will be addressed in more depth in chapter 5.
2. Norm Denzin, *Sociological Methods: A Sourcebook* (New York: McGraw Hill, 1978).
3. On the "new medical pluralism" see Cant and Sharma, *A New Medical Pluralism?*
4. Clifford Geertz, *Local Knowledge* (New York: Basic Books, 1983), 57.
5. For a useful application of Geertz's concepts in the pursuit of a macrosociology see James Bohman, "Habermas, Marxism, and Social Theory: The Case of Pluralism in Critical Social Science," in *Habermas: A Critical Reader,* ed. Peter Dews, 53–86 (Oxford: Blackwell, 1999).

Chapter 1. The Study of Alternative Health

1. David Eisenberg et al., "Unconventional Medicine in the United States," *New England Journal of Medicine* 328 (1993): 246–252 and "Trends in Alternative Medicine Use in the United States, 1990–1997: Results of a Follow-Up National Survey," *Journal of the American Medical Association* 280 (1998):

1569–1575. Another JAMA study showed a somewhat smaller percentage of the U.S. population using alternative medicine. But it also demonstrated that for most people, alternative medicine is a complement, not alternative to conventional medicine. See Benjamin G. Druss, M.D., M.Ph.; Robert A. Rosenheck, M.D., "Association between Use of Conventional Therapies and Conventional Medical Services," JAMA 282 (1999): 651–656. Another survey that compared patients of an alternative health center with a control group of patients, showed that the two groups differed in terms of two variables; the alternative group "lacked confidence in conventional medical treatment" and thought of themselves as more unconventional than the control group. See Katherine J. McGregor and Edmund R. Peay, "The Choice of Alternative Therapy for Health Care: Testing Some Propositions," *Social Science and Medicine* 43 (1996): 1317–1327.

2. Bill Moyers, *Healing and the Mind* (New York: Doubleday, 1993). The book is based on the TV series by the same name.

3. D. Ornish, *Dr. Dean Ornish's Program for Reversing Heart Disease* (New York: Random House, 1990).

4. A. Weil, *Eight Weeks to Optimal Health: A Proven Program for Taking Full Advantage of Your Body's Natural Healing Power* (New York: Knopf, 1997).

5. Among Chopra's many popular books see, D. Chopra, *Quantum Healing: Exploring the Frontiers of Mind-Body Medicine* (New York: Bantam Books, 1989).

6. A good discussion of the history of the NIH Office of Alternative Medicine can be found in Michael S. Goldstein, *Alternative Health Care: Medicine, Miracle, or Mirage?* (Philadelphia: Temple University Press, 1999), 176–184. The OAM has been upgraded to a center and is now the Center for Complementary and Alternative Medicine.

7. I. C. Illich, *Medical Nemesis* (New York: Random House, 1976), 13–36.

8. Also see Rene Dubos, *The Mirage of Health* (Garden City, NY: Doubleday, 1959) and Thomas McKeown, *The Role of Medicine* (Princeton: Princeton University Press, 1979).

9. "The Boom in Medications Bring Rise in Fatal Risks," *New York Times,* June 3, 1999.

10. On the "epidemiological revolution" see Richard Levins, "Is Capitalism a Disease? The Crisis in U.S. Health Care," *Monthly Review* 52 (2000): 8–11.

11. There is now a vast literature on chronic illness in sociology. Here are a few examples, A. L. Strauss and B.G., *Glaser Chronic Illness and the Quality of Life* (St. Louis: Mosby, 1975); *The Experience and Management of Chronic Illness* (Research in the Sociology of Health Care, Vol. 6) (Greenwich, CT: JAI Press, 1987); *Social Science and Medicine* 30 (1990): Special Issue, "Qualitative Research on Chronic Illness"; Kathy Charmaz, *Good Days, Bad Days: The Self in Chronic Illness* (New Brunswick, NJ: Rutgers University Press, 1991).

12. Institute of Medicine, *Emerging Infections: Microbial Threats to Health in the United States* (Washington, DC: National Academy Press, 1992) and Gregory L. Armstrong, M.D., Laura A. Conn, M.P.H., Robert W. Pinner, M.D., "Trends in Infectious Disease Mortality in the United States During the 20th Century," *Journal of the American Medical Association* 281 (1999): 61–66. The return of many infectious diseases and the global transmission of new disease-carrying microbes is the theme of Laurie Garrett, *The Coming Plague* (New York: Farrar, Straus and Giroux, 1994).

13. On the changing cultural meaning of the "immune system" see Emily Martin, *Flexible Bodies: Tracking Immunity in American Culture from the Days of Polio to the Age of AIDS* (Boston: Beacon Press, 1994).

14. The American Cancer Society's website provides data on age adjusted cancer rates since 1930. Progress has been made primarily in the area of diagnosis but only a few forms of cancer have shown significant declines in death rates since 1930. For example, death rates have declined for Hodgkin's disease, testicular cancer, and childhood leukemia but these are the exception not the rule. Death rates for lung and skin cancer are increasing while death rates for stomach, breast, and colon cancer have not significantly changed since 1930. Also see for a discussion and critique of the "cancer war," Robert Proctor, *Cancer Wars: How Politics Shapes What We Know and Don't Know About Cancer* (New York: Basic Books, 1995); Samuel Epstein, M.D., *The Politics of Cancer Revisited* (Fremont Center, NY: East Ridge Press, 1998); R. Moss, The Cancer Industry: The Classic Expose on the Cancer Establishment (New York: Equinox Press, 1996).

15. Robert A. Aronowitz, *Making Sense of Illness: Science, Society, and Disease* (Cambridge: Cambridge University Press, 1998).

16. U. Sharma, *Complementary Medicine Today: Practitioners and Patients* (London: Routledge, 1992); S. Cant and M. Calnan, "On the Margins of the Medical Marketplace? An Exploratory Study of Alternative Practitioners Perceptions," *Sociology of Health and Illness* 12 (1991): 34–51.

17. On the social consequences of chronic illness see Arthur Kleinman, *The Illness Narratives: Suffering, Healing, and the Human Condition* (New York: Basic Books, 1998) and Writing on the *Margin: Discourse between Anthropology and Medicine* (Berkeley: University of California Press, 1995), 95–189.

18. Charmaz, *Good Days, Bad Days,* 257–265.

19. Two excellent overviews of how alternative health resonates with larger cultural shifts in American society can be found in Goldstein, *Alternative Health Care,* 13–39; June S. Lowenberg, *Caring and Responsibility: The Crossroads between Holistic Practice and Traditional Medicine* (Philadelphia: University of Pennsylvania Press, 1989), 53–92.

20. The Boston Women's Health Book Collective, *Our Bodies, Ourselves: For the New Century* (New York: Simon and Schuster, 1998), 29–178.

21. William G. McLoughlin, *Revivals, Awakenings, and Reform: An Essay on Religion and Social Change,* 1607–1977 (Chicago and London: University of Chicago Press, 1978), 179–216.

22. Victor W. Turner, "Communitas: Model and Process," in *The Ritual Process: Structure and Anti-Structure* (Chicago: Aldine, 1969), 131–165.

23. Cant and Sharma, *A New Medical Pluralism?,* 5–9.

24. Ibid., 92.

25. The problem of how to define alternative health is addressed in Walter J. Wardwell, "Alternative Medicine in the United States," *Social Science and Medicine* 38 (1994): 1061–1068. Paul Wolpe regards alternative health as a "heretical movement" that challenges the hegemonic medical discourse. See Paul Root Wolpe, "The Holistic Heresy: Strategies of Ideological Challenge in the Medical Profession," *Social Science and Medicine* 31 (1990): 913–923.

26. See D. T. Jaffe, *The Holistic Perspective. Holistic Health Focus,* p. 3, quoted in Lowenberg, *Caring and Responsibility,* 30.

27. The classic account of the "sick role" in sociological theory comes from Talcott Parsons, *The Social System* (New York: Free Press, 1951), 428–479.

28. The first major text was Robert Ader, David L. Felton, and Nicholas Cohen, eds., *Psychoneuroimmunology,* second edition (San Diego: Academic Press, 1991).

29. Lowenberg, *Caring and Responsibility,* 15–52.

30. Epstein, *The Politics of Cancer, Revisited,* 473–510. A short version of Epstein's argument can be found in Samuel Epstein and Liza Gross, "The High Stakes of Cancer Prevention," *Tikkun,* November/December 2000, 33–39.

31. An overview of alternative cancer treatments can be found in Michael Lerner, *Choices in Healing: Integrating the Best of Conventional and Approaches to Cancer* (Cambridge: MIT Press, 1998).

32. Cant and Sharma, *A New Medical Pluralism?,* 96–100.

33. J. Pickstone, "Ways of Knowing: Towards a Historical Sociology of Science, Technology and Medicine," *British Journal of the History of Science* 26 (1993): 433–58.

34. One of many examples of this evolutionary approach to "folk medicine" is Charles Bundy Wilson, "Notes on Folk-Medicine," *Journal of American Folklore* 21, no. 80 (1908): 68–73.

35. A useful overview and critique of functionalist and psychological approaches to alternative medicine can be found in Bonnie Blair O'Connor, *Healing Traditions: Alternative Medicine and the Health Professions* (Philadelphia: University of Pennsylvania Press, 1995), 41–44.

36. An example of this bias, in which alternative health is judged by the standards of biomedicine, is W. Wardwell, "Alternative Medicine in the United States," *Social Science and Medicine* 38 (1994): 1061–1068.

37. For a useful review of this literature see Cant and Sharma, *A New Medical Pluralism?,* 21–50.

38. Lowenberg, *Caring and Responsibility*, 53–156.

39. Hans A. Baer, *Biomedicine and Alternative Healing Systems in America: Issues of Class, Race, Ethnicity, and Gender* (Madison: University of Wisconsin Press, 2001). Another recent work which adopts the "medical pluralism" perspective is Cant and Sharma, *A New Medical Pluralism?*

40. O'Connor, *Healing Traditions*, 80–108.

41. Arthur Frank, *The Wounded Story Teller: Body, Illness, and Ethics* (Chicago: University of Chicago Press, 1995).

42. Elaine Scarry, *The Body in Pain* (New York: Oxford University Press, 1985).

43. Meredith McGuire, *Ritual Healing in Suburban America* (New Brunswick: Rutgers University Press, 1991).

44. Nicholas J. Fox, *Postmodernism, Sociology, and Health* (Toronto: University of Toronto Press, 1994). Frohock's work on the spiritual dimension of alternative health and the policy implications of the competing philosophies of biomedicine and alternative medicine challenges any notion of objective truth. In this respect his work is part of the postmodern tradition. See Fred M. Frohock, *Healing Powers: Alternative Medicine, Spiritual Communities, and the State* (Chicago: University of Chicago Press, 1992). For a discussion of the nature of "postmodern illness" see David B. Morris, *Illness and Culture in the Postmodern Age* (Berkeley and Los Angeles: University of California Press, 1998).

45. Axel Honneth, "Pluralization and Recognition: On the Self Misunderstanding of Postmodern Social Theorists," in *Between Totalitarianism and Postmodernity,* ed. Peter Beilharz, Gillian Robinson, and John Rundell, 163–172 (Cambridge: MIT Press, 1992).

46. Barry Glassner, "Fit For Postmodern Selfhood," in *Symbolic Interaction and Cultural Studies,* ed. Howard S. Becker and Michael M. McCall, 221 (Chicago: University of Chicago Press, 1990).

47. Glassner, "Fit For Postmodern Selfhood," 228. Also on fitness and wellness see Michael S. Goldstein, *The Health Movement: Promoting Fitness in America* (New York: Twayne, 1992).

48. The term *total social process* comes from T. Adorno, *Negative Dialectics* (New York: Seabury, 1973), 314.

49. A useful collection of essays on the application of Habermas and critical theory to health care issues is, Graham Scambler, ed., *Habermas, Critical Theory, and Health* (London and New York: Routledge, 2001).

50. Max Weber, "Science as a Vocation," in *From Max Weber: Essays in Sociology,* ed. H. H. Gerth and C. W. Mills, 129–156 (New York: Oxford University Press, 1958).

51. Benedict Anderson, *Imagined Communities; Reflections on the Origin and Spread of Nationalism* (London: Verso, 1991) and Eric Hobsbawm and Terence Ranger, eds., *The Invention of Tradition* (Cambridge: Cambridge University Press, 1982).

52. Lowenberg, *Caring and Responsibility*, 53–92.

53. Max Weber, *Protestant Ethic and the Spirit of Capitalism* (New York: Scribner, 1958), 181.

Chapter 2. Biomedicine and the Loss of Meaning

1. A study published in JAMA 1998 estimated that 106,000 hospital patients die and 2.2 million are injured each year by adverse reactions to prescription drugs. The National Association of Chain Drug Stores reports that in 1992, 2.03 billion prescriptions were dispensed in pharmacies. This went up to 2.78 billion in 1998 and it is estimated to be 4 billion in 2005. For a popular discussion of this issue see Sheryl Gay Stolberg "The Boom in Medications Brings Rise in Fatal Risks," *New York Times,* June 3, 1999.
2. On medical errors see Linda T. Kohn, Janet M. Corrigan, and Molla S. Donaldson, editors; Committee on the Quality of Health Care in America, Institute of Medicine, *To Err is Human* (Washington, D.C.: National Academy Press, 2000). The data on mistakes in hospitals can be found in American Hospital Association, Hospital Statistics, Chicago, 1999; Also see "Results of the Medical Practice Study," *New England Journal of Medicine* 324 (1991): 370–376.
3. For a further discussion of how everyday life becomes deritualized see Anthony Giddens, *The Consequences of Modernity* (Stanford: Stanford University Press, 1990), 36–40.
4. See Arthur Kleinman, "What is Specific to Biomedicine?" in *Writing at the Margins,* 21–40.
5. Paul Starr, *The Social Transformation of American Medicine* (New York: Basic Books, 1982), 30–78.
6. Robert Fuller, *Alternative Medicine and American Religious Life* (New York: Oxford University Press, 1989); James C. Whorton, *Crusaders for Fitness* (Princeton: Princeton University Press, 1982); Henri Ellenberger, *The Discovery of the Unconscious* (New York: Basic Books, 1970); Donald Meyer, *The Positive Thinkers: Religion as Pop Psychology from Mary Barker Eddy to Oral Roberts* (New York: Pantheon Books, 1980).
7. Baer, *Biomedicine and Alternative Healing Systems in America,* 13.
8. Ibid., 17–20.
9. Ann Braude, *Radical Spirits: Spiritualism and Women's Rights in Nineteenth-Century America* (Boston: Beacon Press, 1989).
10. Starr, *The Social Transformation of Medicine,* 109–144.
11. Jürgen Habermas, *The Theory of Communicative Action; Reason and the Rationalization of Society, Vol. 1* (Boston: Beacon Press, 1984), 238–242 and *The Theory of Communicative Action: Lifeworld and System, Vol. 2* (Boston: Beacon Press, 1987), 327–331.
12. Starr, *The Social Transformation of American Medicine,* 79–144.

13. Quoted in Hans A. Baer, "The American Dominative Medical System as a Reflection of Social Relations in the Larger Society," *Social Science and Medicine* 28 (1989): 1106.
14. Steffie Woolhandler and David U. Himmelstein, "Ideology in Medical Science: Class in the Clinic," *Social Science and Medicine* 28 (1989): 1206.
15. Epstein and Gross, "The High Stakes of Cancer Prevention," 37–38.
16. Levins, "Is Capitalism a Disease?" 16.
17. Andre Gorz, *Paths to Paradise: On the Liberation from Work.* (Boston: South End Press, 1985), 22–24.
18. Habermas, *The Theory of Communicative Action, Vol. 1,* 113–152 and Alfred Schutz, *Collected Papers 1: The Problem of Social Reality,* ed. M. Natanson (The Hague: Kluwer Academic Publishers, 1962).
19. We derive this Heideggerian analysis from Lorenzo C. Simpson, *Technology, Time, and the Conversations of Modernity* (New York: Routledge, 1995), 75–94.
20. Martin Heidegger, "The Age of the World Picture," in *The Question Concerning Technology and Other Essays* (New York: Harper and Row, 1977), 103, 123. For interesting discussions of Heidegger's idea of world picture see Malcolm Bull, *Seeing Things Hidden: Apocalypse, Vision, and Totality* (London: Verso, 2000), 173–186.
21. Maeve Cooke, *Language and Reason: A Study of Habermas's Pragmatics* (Cambridge: MIT Press, 1997), 15–27.
22. This idea of Benjamin is emphasized in Habermas's essay, "Walter Benjamin: Consciousness Raising or Rescuing Critique," in *Philosophical-Political Profiles* (Cambridge: MIT Press, 1983), 156.
23. Habermas, "Walter Benjamin: Consciousness Raising or Rescuing Critique?" 156.
24. Byron J. Good, *Medicine, Rationality, and Experience: An Anthropological Perspective* (Cambridge: Cambridge University Press, 1994), 65–87 Also for an interesting account of medical communication in the context of a hospital setting see Lillian R. Furst, *Between Doctors and Patients* (Charlottesville: University Press of Virginia, 1998), 217–251.
25. Good, *Medicine, Rationality, and Experience,* 79.
26. Lewis Mehl-Madrona, M.D., *Coyote Medicine* (New York: Scribner, 1997), 29.
27. For a collection of studies on doctor-patient communication see Mack Lipkin Jr., Samuel M. Putnam, and Aaron Lazare, eds.; Allen Keller, Terri Klein, and P. Kay Williams, asst. eds., *The Medical Interview; Clinical Care, Education, and Research* (New York: Springer Verlag, 1995). Also see Elliot Mishler, *The Discourse of Medicine: Dialectics of Medical Interviews* (Norwood, NJ: Ablex, 1986).
28. Jennie Papay, Garth Williams, Tori Gabriel, and Carol Thames, "Exploring the Meaning and Dissatisfaction with Healthcare, The Importance of Personal Identity Threat," *Sociology of Health and Illness* 21 (1999): 95–121.

29. Mishler, *The Discourse of Medicine: Dialectics of Medical Interviews*. Also see Graham Scambler, "Habermas and the Power of Medical Expertise," in *Sociological Theory and Medical Sociology*, 165–193.

30. Cheryl Mattingly, "In Search of the Good: Narrative Reasoning in Clinical Practice," *Medical Anthropology Quarterly* 12, no. 3 (1998): 279–280.

31. Furst, *Between Doctors and Patients*, 8.

32. Habermas, *The Theory of Communicative Action, Vol. 2*, 374–403.

33. S. Lukes, *Power: A Radical View* (London: Macmillan, 1974).

34. Renee R. Anspach, "Notes on the Sociology of Medical Discourse: The Language of Case Presentation," *Journal of Health and Social Behavior* 29 (1988): 357–375.

35. Ibid., 367.

36. Ibid., 366.

37. H. Graham and A. Oakley, "Competing Ideologies of Reproduction: Medical and Maternal Perspectives on Pregnancy," in *Women, Health, and Reproduction*, ed. H. Roberts (London: Routledge, 1981).

38. Ibid., 183.

39. Arthur Frank, *The Wounded Story Teller*, 172–176.

40. Elaine Scarry, *The Body in Pain*.

41. See the following on professionalization within alternative medicine: Maria J. Verhoff and Lloyd R. Sutherland, "General Practitioners Assessment of and Interest in Alternative Medicine in Canada," *Social Science and Medicine* 41 (1995): 511–515; Paul Root Wolpe, "The Maintenance of Professional Authority: Acupuncture and the American Physician," *Social Problems* 32 (1985): 409–421; Hans A. Baer, Cindy Jen, Lucia M. Tanassi, Christopher Tsia, and Helen Wahbeth, "The Drive for Professionalization in Acupuncture: A Preliminary View from the San Francisco Bay Area," *Social Science and Medicine* 46 (1997): 533–537; Philip Tovey, "Contingent legitimacy: U.K. Alternative Practitioners and Inter-Sectoral Acceptance," *Social Science and Medicine* 45 (1997): 1129–1133.

42. O'Connor, *Healing Traditions*, 109–160.

43. Giddens, *The Consequences of Modernity*, 36–40.

44. An interesting discussion of this phenomenon from a Jungian perspective can be found in Andrew Samuel, *The Political Psyche* (London and New York: Routledge, 1993).

Chapter 3. Between the Aura and the Commodity

1. Richard Wolin, *Walter Benjamin: An Aesthetic of Redemption* (Berkeley: University of California Press, 1994), 1–28.

2. Walter Benjamin, *Illuminations* (New York: Schocken, 1968), 83–109.

3. Weber, *Science as a Vocation*, 129–156.

4. Benjamin, *Illuminations*, 257.

5. Ibid., 263.

6. Walter Benjamin, *Origin of German Tragic Drama* (London: New Left Books, 1977).

7. Habermas, *Philosophical-Political Profiles,* 129–165.

8. Benjamin, *Illuminations,* 217–251.

9. Walter Benjamin, *Reflections* (New York: Schocken, 1978), 314–337 and Habermas, *Philosophical-Political Profiles,* 146–150.

10. Benjamin, *Illuminations,* 155–194 and *Reflections,* 333–334.

11. On Benjamin's theory of language see Susan A. Handelman, *Fragments of Redemption: Jewish Thought and Literary Theory in Benjamin, Scholem, and Levinas* (Bloomington: Indiana University Press, 1991), 15–61.

12. Warren J. Belasco, *Appetite for Change: How the Counterculture Took on the Food Industry* (Ithaca and London: Cornell University Press, 1993), 72.

13. Quoted in Belasco, 23.

14. On New Age health practices and the New Age movement see, J. A. English-Lueck, *Health in the New Age: A Study of California Holistic Practices* (Albuquerque: University of New Mexico Press, 1990) and K. B. Alster, *The Holistic Health Movement* (Tuscaloosa: University of Alabama Press, 1989).

15. Fuller, *Alternative Medicine and American Religious Life,* 35–37.

16. Ibid., 113.

17. Terry Eagleton, *Walter Benjamin: Or Toward A Revolutionary Criticism* (London: Verso, 1981), 29.

18. On the culture of consumption see Stuart Ewen, *Captains of Consciousness: Advertising and the Roots of the Consumer Culture* (New York: McGraw-Hill, 1976); Richard Wightman Fox and T. J. Lears, eds., *The Culture of Consumption: Critical Essays in American History: 1880–1980* (New York: Pantheon, 1983); Jackson Lears, *Fables of Abundance: A Cultural History of Advertising in America* (New York: Harper Collins, 1994); Roland Marchland, *Advertising and the American Dream: Making the Way for Modernity, 1920–1940* (Berkeley: University of California Press, 1986); Michael Schudson, *Advertising: The Uneasy Persuasion: Its Dubious Impact on American Society* (New York: Basic Books, 1984).

19. On the active use people make of commodities when they reembed them in everyday life see John Fiske, *Reading the Popular* (Boston: Unwin Hyman, 1989).

20. Benjamin, *Illuminations,* 155–200.

21. Studies of drug-taking behavior are in their infancy. One such study examines "the personal logics underlying medicine taking" and examines medicine-related practice in a larger social and political-economic perspective. See Nancy Vuckovic and Mark Nichter, "Changing Patterns of Pharmaceutical Practice in the United States," *Social Science and Medicine* 44 (1997): 1285–1302.

22. *Better Homes and Gardens,* April 1998.

23. Jean Paul Sartre, *The Critique of Dialectical Reason, Vol. 1* (London: New Left Books, 1976), 256–306.

24. On the food co-op movement see Craig Cox, *Storefront Revolution: Food Co-ops and the Counterculture* (New Brunswick, NJ.: Rutgers University Press, 1994).

25. Habermas, *A Berlin Republic: Writings on Germany* (Translated by Steven Rendall) (Lincoln: University of Nebraska Press, 1997), 122–127.

26. Mehl-Madrona, *Coyote Medicine*.

27. Barrington Moore Jr., *Social Origins of Dictatorship and Democracy* (Boston: Beacon, 1966), 509–523.

28. Alberto Melucci, *Challenging Codes: Collective Action in the Information Age* (Cambridge: Cambridge University Press, 1996), 104.

29. Eric Wolf, *Peasant Wars of the Twentieth Century* (New York: Harper, 1969).

30. Fred Evans, "Voices of Chiapas: The Zapatistas, Bakhtin, and Human Rights," *Philosophy Today* 42 (2000): 196–210.

31. Adolfo Gilly, "Chiapas and the Rebellion of the Enchanted World," in *Rural Revolt in Mexico,* ed. Daniel Nugent, 261–334 (Durham: Duke University Press, 1998). The passage cited is on 327.

32. Alberto Melucci, *Nomads of the Present: Social Movements and Individual Needs in Contemporary Society* (Philadelphia: Temple University Press, 1989), 120.

33. Melucci, *Challenging Codes,* 97–113.

34. Robert N. Proctor, *The Nazi War on Cancer* (Princeton: Princeton University Press, 1999).

35. Mark Neocleous, *Fascism* (Minneapolis: University of Minnesota, 1997), 75–88.

36. On the problematic use of the natural see, Anthony Giddens, *Beyond Left and Right: The Future of Radical Politics* (Stanford: Stanford University Press, 1994), 208–212 and Andrew Ross, "New Age Technoculture," in *Cultural Studies,* ed. Lawrence Grossberg, Cary Nelson, and Paula Treichler, 531–555 (New York: Routledge, 1992).

Chapter 4. Technologies of the Self

1. A. MacGregor and E. Peay "The Choice of Alternative Therapy for Health Care," *Social Science and Medicine* 43 (1996): 1317–1327; A. Furnham and C. Smith, "Choosing Alternative Medicine: A Comparison of the Patients Visiting a GP and a Homeopath," *Social Science and Medicine* 26 (1988): 685–687.

2. While Eisenberg's survey shows that most users of alternative health products and services combine these with conventional medicine, his sample includes the large group of people who have had some contact with alternative medicine. In this chapter we are concerned with the chronically ill who are committed to alternative health and have typically been dissatisfied with their treatment from conventional medicine.

3. Nathan Leites and Charles Wolf Jr., *Rebellion and Authority: An Analytic Essay on Insurgent Conflicts* (Chicago: Markham, 1970); Mancur Olson, *The Logic of Collective Action* (Cambridge: MIT Press, 1965).

4. Barrington Moore, *Injustice: The Social Basis of Obedience and Revolt* (White Plains, NY: M.E. Sharpe, 1978); E. P. Thompson, *The Making of the English Working Class* (New York: Random House, 1966).

5. On the sociology of the body see Mike Featherstone, "The Body in Consumer Culture," *Theory, Culture, and Society* 8 (1982): 18–33; Bryan Turner, *The Body and Society: Explorations in Social Theory* (Oxford: Blackwell, 1984) and *Regulating Bodies: Essays in Medical Sociology* (London: Routledge, 1992).

6. Michel Foucault, *The History of Sexuality: Vol. 1: Introduction* (New York: Random House, 1978); *The History of Sexuality: Vol. 2: The Use of Pleasure* (New York: Random House, 1983); *The History of Sexuality: Vol. 3: The Care of the Self* (New York: Random House, 1986).

7. Jürgen Habermas, *The Philosophical Discourse of Modernity* (Cambridge: MIT Press, 1987), 238–265.

8. Michel Foucault, *Interviews and Other Writings* (New York: Routledge, 1988), 119–120.

9. Michel Foucault, *The History of Sexuality: Vol. 2*. Also see Luther Martin, Huck Butman, and Patrick H. Hutton, *Technologies of the Self: A Seminar with Michel Foucault* (Amherst: University of Massachusetts Press, 1988).

10. Anne E. Frahm with David J. Frahm, *A Cancer Battle Plan: Six Strategies for Beating Cancer, from a Recovered "Hopeless Case"* (New York: Jeremy P. Tarcher/Putnam, 1997).

11. Zygmunt Bauman, "A Sociological Theory of Postmodernity," in *Thesis Eleven Reader,* ed. Peter Beiharz, Gillian Robinson, and John Rundell (Cambridge: MIT Press, 1992); Habermas, *The Philosophical Discourse of Modernity;* Axel Honneth, "Pluralization and Recognition: On the Self-Misunderstanding of Postmodern Social Theorist," in *Between Totalitarianism and Postmodernity,* ed. Peter Beiharz, Gillian Robinson, and John Rundell, 163–172 (Cambridge: MIT Press, 1992); Scott Lash, *Sociology of Postmodernism* (London: Routledge, 1990).

12. Michael Shannon, "A Quartet for Our Times," *New Left Review* 201 (1993): 101–112. See 107–108.

13. Edward Said, *Musical Elaborations* (New York: Columbia University Press, 1991).

14. On aesthetic theory see, Theodor W. Adorno, *Aesthetic Theory,* trans. C. Lendardt, (London: Routledge, 1984); Terry Eagleton, *The Ideology of the Aesthetic* (Oxford: Blackwell, 1990); Stefan Morawski, *Inquiries into the Fundamentals of Aesthetics* (Cambridge: Harvard University Press, 1974); Charles Taylor, *Hegel* (Cambridge: MIT Press, 1977), 22–29.

15. For a discussion of the body "as the focal point of self-construction" from a phenomenological perspective see Robin Saltonstall, "Healthy Bodies, Social Bodies: Men's and Women's Concepts and Practices of Health in Everyday Life," *Social Science and Medicine* 36 (1993): 7–14.

16. Melucci, *Challenging Codes,* 105.
17. Peter Dews, *The Limits of Disenchantment: Essays on Contemporary European Philosophy* (London: Verso, 1995); Alberto Melucci, *Nomads of the Present,* 119–126.
18. Fuller, *Alternative Medicine and American Religious Life,* 38–65.
19. Taylor, *Hegel.*
20. This line is from a T. S. Eliot poem ("Burnt Norton").
21. Nancy Fraser, *Justice Interruptus: Critical Reflection on the Postsocialist Condition* (New York: Routledge, 1997), 70.
22. Ibid., 80–85.
23. Ibid., 69–98.

Chapter 5. New Social Movements

1. See the following on new social movements: Steven Buechler, "New Social Movement Theories," *The Sociological Quarterly* 36 (1995): 441–464; Jean L. Cohen, "Strategy or Identity: New Theoretical Paradigms and Contemporary Social Movements," *Social Research* 52 (1985): 663–716; Klaus Eder, "A New Social Movement?" *Telos* 52 (1982): 5–20; Enrique Larana, Hank Johnston, and Joseph Gusfield, eds., *New Social Movements: From Ideology to Identity* (Philadelphia: Temple University Press, 1994); Claus Offe, "New Social Movements: Challenging the Boundaries of Institutional Politics," *Social Research* 52 (1985): 817–868; Alberto Melucci, "The New Social Movements: A Theoretical Approach," *Social Science Information* 19 (1980): 199–226; "The New Social Movement Revisited: Reflections on a Sociological Misunderstanding," in Lewis Maheu, ed., *Social Movements and Social Classes,* 107–119 (London: Sage, 1995).
2. Habermas, *The Theory of Communicative Action, Vols. 1 and 2.*
3. Jürgen Habermas. *Legitimation Crisis* (Boston: Beacon Press, 1973).
4. Habermas, *The Theory of Communicative Action, Vol. 2,* 356–373. The discussion of family law is on 368. Also see James Bohman, *The New Philosophy of Social Science* (Cambridge: MIT Press, 1991), 183–185.
5. Habermas, *The Theory of Communicative Action, Vol. 2,* 394.
6. Melucci, *Nomads of the Present,* 18.
7. Alberto Melucci, "The Process of Collective Identity," 41–63 in Hank Johnston and Bert Klandermans, eds., *Social Movements and Culture* (Minneapolis: University of Minnesota Press, 1995).
8. On studies of submerged new social movements networks see Carol Mueller, "Conflict Networks and the Origins of Women's Liberation," in *New Social Movements,* 234–263; Verta Taylor and Nancy E. Whittier, "Collective Identity in Social Movement Communities: Lesbian Feminist Mobilization," in *Frontiers in Social Movement Theory,* ed. Aldon D. Morris and Carol McClung Mueller, 104–129, (New Haven: Yale University Press,

1992); Verta Taylor, "Social Movement Continuity: The Women's Movement in Abeyance," *American Sociological Review* 54 (1989): 761–775.

9. Melucci, *Nomads of the Present,* 29.

10. Ibid., 58–80.

11. Claus Offe, *Disorganized Capitalism* (Cambridge: MIT Press, 1985).

12. Jürgen Habermas, *The New Conservatism: Cultural Criticism and the Historians' Debate* (Cambridge: MIT Press, 1989), 66–67.

13. James Davidson Hunter, *Culture Wars: The Struggle to Define America* (New York: Basic Books, 1991).

14. Ray Oldenburg, *The Great Good Places: Cafes, Coffee Shops, Community Centers, Beauty Parlors, General Stores, Bars, Hangouts and How they Get You Through the Day* (New York: Paragon House, 1985).

15. Sara Evans, *Personal Politics: The Roots of Women's Liberation in the Civil Rights Movement and New Left* (New York: Random House, 1980).

16. Ivan Illich, *Toward a History of Needs* (Berkeley: Heyday, 1977).

17. A. Relman, "The Medical-Industrial Complex," *New England Journal of Medicine* 303 (1980): 963–970.

18. On prefigurative politics see Sara Evans and Harry Boyte, *Free Spaces* (New York: Harper and Row, 1986).

19. On postmaterial values see Ronald Inglehart, *The Silent Revolution: Changing Values and Political Styles among Western Publics* (Princeton: Princeton University Press, 1977).

20. The classic study was directed by Dr. Michael Marmont, director of the International Center for Health and Society at University College London. It tracked mortality rates over ten years for 17,530 male civil service employees. A twenty-five year followup of the Whitehall subjects was published in 1996 and showed an even closer relationship between socioeconomic status and mortality.

21. Buechler provides a very valuable overview and critique of new social movement theory in his latest book. He is also critical of the assertion among earlier new social movement theorists that class-based politics is a thing of the past. See, Steven M. Buechler, *Social Movements in Advanced Capitalism; The Political Economy and Cultural Construction of Social Activism* (New York: Oxford University Press, 2000), 123–127.

22. Our finding in this respect is similar to Goldstein's research on the differences between holistic and conventional doctors. See Michael Goldstein, Dennis T. Jaffe, Dale Garell, and Ruth Ellen Berkem "Holistic Physicians and Family Practitioners: Similarities, Differences, and Implications for Health Policy," *Urban Life* 14 (1985): 316–344. Also see Adrian Furnham and Chris Smith, "Choosing Alternative Medicine: A Comparison of the Beliefs of Patients Visiting a General Practitioner and a Homeopath," *Social Science and Medicine* 26 (1988): 685–689.

23. An interesting discussion of the animal rights movement and its relationship to left movements can be found in Ted Benton and Simon

Redfearn, "The Politics of Animal Rights—Where is the Left?" *New Left Review* 215 (1996): 43–58.

24. We note here that while our data strongly support our claims concerning the collective identity of these two alternative health networks and their character as new social movement networks, our claim concerning the connections between this movement and others is strongly suggested by our data but not entirely demonstrated. Instead, we would see this claim as a hypothesis generated by our data, which has some support, but which also would require further study.

25. Cant and Sharma report a correlation between level of professionalization (full-time training, scientifically oriented, higher salaries, formal credentials, unity among practitioners) in alternative health and the percentage of men who are practitioners. For example, in fields such as chiropractic, which is far more professionalized than reflexology, there are more men. This is consistent with our explanation that technologies of the self are a gendered practice but it's also consistent with the reality for many professional women that they must combine work and family responsibilities. The less professionalized branches of alternative health offer more opportunities for part-time work but these less professionalized therapies are also closer to the lifeworlds of patients. See Cant and Sharma, *A New Medical Pluralism?*, 75.

Chapter 6. From Alternative to Complementary Medicine

1. Melucci, *Nomads of the Present* and *Challenging Codes.*
2. Habermas, *The Theory of Communicative Action, Vol. 2*, 113–199.
3. Our argument runs counter to both the earlier versions of resource mobilization theory, which emphasized social movement organization, and to Piven and Cloward's highly influential work, *Poor Peoples Movements: Why They Succeed, How They Fail* (New York: Vintage, 1979), which argued that social movement organization leads to the co-optation of movements.
4. Miriam S. Wetzel, Ph.D., David M. Eisenberg, M.D., Ted J. Kaptchuk, O.M.D., "Courses Involving Complementary and Alternative Medicine at US Medical Schools," *JAMA* 280 (1998): 784–787. Also see the letters in response to this article, especially Michael Carlston, M.D., who noted that presenting courses on alternative or complementary medicine does not indicate advocacy and Dr. Sergeant who is "appalled" at the results of the survey showing widespread adoption of courses on alternative medicine. For Dr. Sergeant, alternative medicine is "pseudoscience." *JAMA* 281 (1999).
5. Sidney Tarrow, *Power in Movement: Social Movements, Collective Action, and Politics* (Cambridge: Cambridge University Press, 1994).

6. R. Ader and D. L. Felton, *Psychoneuroimmunology,* ed. N. Cohen, 2nd edition (Orlando: Academic Press, 1991); D. Sobel, "Rethinking Medicine: Improving Health Outcomes with Cost-Effective Intervention," *Psychosomatic Medicine* 57 (1995): 234–244; J. A. Turner, R. A. Deyo, J. D. Loeser, M. Von Korff, W. E. Fordyce, "The Importance of Placebo Effects in Pain Treatment and Research," *JAMA* 271 (1994): 1609–1614; National Institutes of Health Technology Assessment Panel, "Integration of Behavioral and Relaxation Approaches Into the Treatment of Chronic Pain and Insomnia," *JAMA* 276 (1996): 313–318. A review of some of this literature, especially recent research on the health benefits of prayer, can be found in Goldstein, *Alternative Health Care,* 13–39.

7. Differences between the approaches of Western biomedicine and more holistic approaches in China and other health systems is discussed in Kleinman, *The Illness Narratives,* 100–120 and *Writing at the Margin,* 95–119.

8. On evidence-based medicine see Daniel J. Friedland, *Evidence-Based Medicine: A Framework for Clinical Practice* (New York: McGraw-Hill, 1998); D. L. Sackett, W. M. Rosenberg, J. A. Gray, R. B. Haynes, W. S. Richardson, "Evidence Based Medicine: What It Is and What It Isn't," *British Medical Journal* 312 (1996): 71–72.

9. Goldstein, *Alternative Health Care,* 33. There is evidence of multiple responses to alternative medicine by various groups of M.D.s. On the one hand there is a kind of backlash against alternative medicine, with claims that it is not scientific and demands that it be subjected to the randomized clinical trial. On the other hand, there is some evidence that many general practitioners use some alternative therapies and have some sympathy for alternative medicine. See Cant and Sharma, *A New Medical Pluralism?,* 96–100.

10. A recent editorial in JAMA cautions against "the rush to embrace a new integration of alternative and conventional medicine. " Interestingly enough, in addition to the usual concerns about the lack of scientific support for alternative modalities and the lack of professional training of alternative practitioners, the editorial also observes that what is most useful in alternative medicine might get lost if it is fully integrated—primarily alternative health's emphasis on self-care and health promotion (rather than pathogenesis). In other words, there are "risks of embracing alternative medicine" and "risks of conventionalizing alternative medicine." Nevertheless, the article maintains that alternative medicine is "here is to stay." See "Alternative Medicine—Learning from the Past, Examining the Present, Advancing to the Future," *JAMA* 280 (1998): 1615–1618.

11. This is consistent with Cant and Sharma's review of the limited literature on the integration of alternative and biomedicine in the West. It appears that this integration does little to challenge the dominance of biomedicine. See Cant and Sharma, *A New Medical Pluralism?,* 157–185.

Conclusion

1. Richard Rorty, *Philosophy and the Mirror of Nature* (Princeton: Princeton University Press, 1979).
2. Jean-Francois Lyotard, *The Postmodern Condition: A Report on Knowledge* (Minneapolis: University of Minnesota Press, 1984).
3. Axel Honneth, *The Struggle for Recognition: The Moral Grammar of Social Conflicts* (Cambridge: MIT Press, 1996), 72.
4. Sartre, *The Critique of Dialectical Reason,* 112–121.
5. Jürgen Habermas, "Modernity vs. Postmodernity," *New German Critique* 22 (1981): 3–18. This article presents the most condensed statement of the problem of mediation that is the central theme of many of Habermas's works.
6. Joseph Schumpeter, *The History of Economic Analysis* (New York: Oxford University Press, 1954), 41.
7. Herman E. Daly, *Beyond Growth: The Economics of Sustainable Development* (Boston: Beacon, 1996), 27–28 and Herman Daly and John B. Cobb Jr., *For the Common Good* (Boston:Beacon, 1989), 25–97.
8. More than forty insurance companies offer at least partial reimbursement for Dean Ornish's dietary regime for heart disease. See Goldstein, *Alternative Health Care,* 209.
9. The National Center for Complementary and Alternative Medicine had a 69 million dollar budget in 2000.
10. Joseph A. Kotarba and Pamela Bentley, "Workplace Wellness Participation and the Becoming of Self," *Social Science and Medicine* 26 (1988): 551–558; Jacqui Alexander, "The Ideological Construction of Risk: An Analysis of Corporate Health Promotion in the 1980's," *Social Science and Medicine* 26 (1988): 559–567; Roberta B. Hollander and Joseph J. Lengermann, "Corporate Characteristics and Worksite Health Promotion Programs: Survey Findings from Fortune 5000 Companies," *Social Science and Medicine* 26 (1988): 491–501.
11. Susan Sontag, *Illness as Metaphor* (New York: Farrar, Straus and Giroux, 1977).
12. Robert D. Putnam, *Bowling Alone: The Collapse and Revival of American Community* (New York: Simon and Schuster, 2000), 93–133.
13. On the Christian Right's extensive subculture see Sarah Diamond, *Not by Politics Alone: The Enduring Influence of the Christian Right* (New York: Guilford, 2000); Christian Smith and Michael Emerson, *American Evangelicalism: Embattled and Thriving* (Chicago: University of Chicago Press, 1998); Justin Watson, *The Christian Coalition: Dreams of Restoration, Demands for Recognition* (New York: St. Martin's,1997).
14. Putnam, *Bowling Alone,* 148–180. For a similar perspective on self-help groups or what Wuthnow calls the "small group movement" see Robert Wuthnow, *Sharing the Journey: Support Groups and America's New Quest for Community* (New York: Free Press, 1994).

15. Putnam, *Bowling Alone,* 22–24.
16. James P. Burke, Ph.D., Ken Williams, M.S., Sharon P. Gaskill, M.P.H., Helen P. Hazuda, Ph.D., Steven M. Hafner, M.D., Michael P. Stern, M.D., "Rapid Rise in the Incidence of Type 2 Diabetes From 1987 to 1996," *Archives of Internal Medicine* 159 (1999): 1450–1456; David Thompson, Ph.D., John Edelsberg, M.D., M.P.H., Graham A. Colditz, M.D., Dr.P.H., Amy P. Bird, Gerry Oster, Ph.D., "Lifetime Health and Economic Consequences of Obesity," *Archives of Internal Medicine* 159 (1999): 2177–2183; Frederick L. Brancati, M.D., M.H.S., W.H. Linda Kao, Ph.D., Aaron R. Folsom, M.D., M.P.H., Robert L. Watson, D.V.M., Ph.D., M.P.H., Moyses Szklo, M.D., Dr.P.H., "Incident Type 2 Diabetes Mellitus in African American and White Adults," JAMA 283 (2000): 2253–2259; Frederick l. Brancati, M.D., M.H.S., Mae-Yuh Wang, Ph.D., Lucy A. Mead, Sc.M., Kung Yee Laing, Ph.D., Michael J. Klang, M.D., M.P.H., "Body Weight Patterns From 20 to 49 Years of Age and Subsequent Risk for Diabetes Mellitus," *Archives of Internal Medicine* 159 (1999): 957–963.
17. Lewin, "Is Capitalism a Disease?" 15–23.
18. Aronowitz, *Making Sense of Illness,* 111–165.
19. Turner, *Regulating Bodies,* 125–150; D. Porter and R. Porter, "What Was Social Medicine? An Historiographic Essay," *Journal of Historical Sociology* 1 (1988): 90–106.
20. A critical assessment of the Genome Project can be found in Richard Lewontin, *It Ain't Necessarily So: The Dream of the Human Genome Project and Other Illusions* (New York: New York Review of Books, 2000).
21. Cant and Sharma, *A New Medical Pluralism?,* 197–199.
22. On the environmental justice movement see, Andrew Szaz, *Ecopopulism: Toxic Waste and the Movement for Environmental Justice (Social Movements, Protest, and Contention,* Vol.1) (Minneapolis: University of Minnesota Press, 1994).

Index

Acidophilus, 106
Activism: grassroots, 2; social, 1
Acupuncture, 74, 86, 87, 112; traditional, 7, 59, 85
Adorno, T., 90
Aesthetic practice, 101, 102
Aesthetic project: alternative health regimes and, 103–105, 109–114; goals of, 105; negative/positive freedom and, 109; self-perfection and, 105
Aesthetics: politics and, 114–121
Agency: modern notion of, 92; potential for, 92
Agriculture: chemicals/pesticides in, 6; natural, 70; organic, 70, 82; sustainable, 5
AIDS, 19, 61, 151; conventional treatment and, 18
Allergies, 27, 63; conventional treatment and, 18
Alternative health: aura and, 67–72; biblical teachings and, 22, 81, 91, 100; in capitalist systems, 35; chronic illness and, 20; classical

aesthetic project and, 15, 25, 109–114; commodified dimension, 77–80, 96; conflicts within, 22; costs of, 17; as cottage industry, 143; creation of new modes of interaction in, 38; credentialization and, 59, 61, 185; as cultural laboratory, 36, 127, 155; defining, 21–29; dual movement character, 156, 157; ecological conception of body, 23; emphasis on change in living, 20; emphasis on holism, 22–24; etiology of disease and, 28; existence on variety of levels of power, 31; gender and, 87; goals, 11; institutionalization of, 156–158, 178–181; integration into dominant health care system, 157–181; language of, 70; legitimacy of, 1; low-tech care in, 24; mediation of expertise in, 58–62; memory inscription in, 37; metaphysical traditions, 22; micro politics of, 101, 188–192; middle

219

common concerns and, 115; information sharing and, 118; state related meanings, 115
Putnam, Robert, 192

Quimby, Phineas, 43

Radiation, 3
Rationality: communicative, 125; crisis, 125; instrumental, 70, 124
Rationalization: in contemporary society, 33; extent to norms not predecided by tradition, 124; of lifeworld, 55, 193; meaningless experiences in, 62; process of, 62; societal, 62, 67; system, 124
Reenchantment: desire for, 65, 73
Reiki, 7, 62
Rejuvenation, 100, 104, 105, 106, 107
Religion: "aesthetic Protestantism," 72; authoritarian character of, 73; critiques of, 73; progressive, 2; prohibitions in, 73
Remedies: herbal, 148; natural, 11, 44, 145
Right, political, 4
Routines, 63

Said, Edward, 109
Scarry, Elaine, 32, 58
School of Holistic Theology, 22
Self: care, 15, 28, 36, 38, 98, 99; creation, 109; description, 11; healing, 24, 25; help, 4, 20; identity, 20, 33; mastery of, 183, 185; perfection, 75, 102; preoccupation with, 2; realization, 126; in relation to illness, 63; transformation, 34, 57, 98
Self, technologies of, 15, 99–122, 183. *See also* Alternative health regimes; alternative health and, 61; autonomous from power regimes, 102; detoxification and, 103–104; gendered practice of,

152; mastery of protocols and, 61; pursuit of knowledge in, 185; rejuvenation and, 104, 105; self-directed, 102
Shamanism, 32, 82
Shiatsu, 7
Social: action, 79, 184; activism, 1; change, 10, 34, 36, 184; class, 145; identity, 78; integration, 48; interaction, 49, 51; justice, 14; movements, 1, 9, 11, 16, 35, 36, 39, 92, 95, 110; pathologies, 55; practices, 63; process, 35, 191; regeneration, 34; rituals, 79; transformation, 114, 121, 185
Social capital: alternative health and, 192; decline in, 192; social movements and, 192
Society: as age of the world picture, 49; changes in relationship to lifeworld through, 49–50; critical theory of, 35; developmental logic of, 124; material reproduction of, 124; meaning in, 15; medicalization of, 11; reflection on the past by, 50; traditional, 11–12, 69
Solomon, Maureen, 6, 61
Sontag, Susan, 192
Spiritualism, 44, 72, 73
Spirituality: alternative health and, 72–77; in alternative health holistic networks, 74; Eastern, 1, 2, 21, 84; importance of, 72; Native American, 21; New Age, 1, 63; as path of healing, 21 the
State: alternative health and, 115; challenges to, 38; legitimacy of, 125; licensing by, 117; meanings of public life and, 115; recognition of alternative health therapies by, 59; regulatory functions, 38; subsidies for biomedicine, 46; suppression of information by, 115–116